The key to being blessed begins with believing that you are.

The key to seeing miracles begins with believing that you will.

And the key to Radiating Hope begins with believing in the brightness of your light.

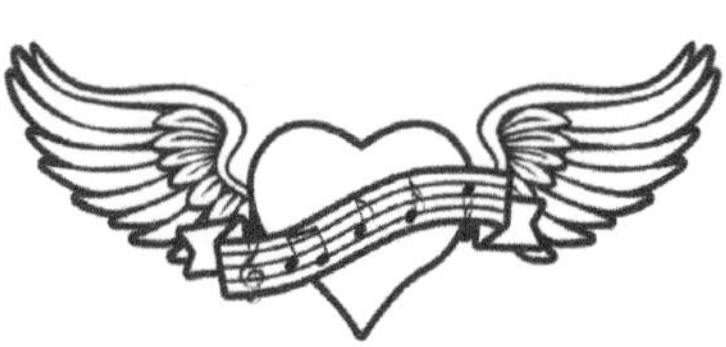

Testimonials

Janie Lidey puts all of her heart into everything she does. Her songs, spirit and writing stand out in profound and impactful ways. She has made a difference in the world around her and the lives of all who know her.

~ John Carter Cash ~
Singer-Songwriter, Author, Producer

I was driving to my oncology appointment on a rainy day and feeling such a lack of hope. I put in Janie Lidey's CD and all of a sudden it was like a bright sunny day and I was filled with hope and inspiration.

~ Carey McLean ~
Innovation Software Engineer and Cancer Survivor

Janie Lidey inspires me to live my best life. To enjoy the simple things that we take for granted.
To realize that there is more in this world than just ourselves and that everyday is special. Just like her!

~ Bobby Rymer ~
Partner/General Manager,
Writer's Den Music Group, Nashville, Tennessee

Janie's words and music move my soul into a peaceful state.

~ Linda Martinez ~
Cancer Survivor

Janie Lidey has done it again. In Radiating Hope ~ Cancer Unplugged, Janie infuses hope, love and light into her readers through her amazing stories and inspirational songs. You don't have to be a cancer survivor for this book to richly bless your life.

~ Craig Duswalt ~
Keynote Speaker, Best-Selling Author, Podcaster,
and Creator of the brands, *RockStar Marketing*
and *Rock Your Life* www.CraigDuswalt.com

Janie Lidey is truly a blessing to all who know her beautiful voice, songs and spirit. I thank God every day for this angel! When I count my blessings, Janie is number one."

~ Mary Loving ~
Director Corporate Travel and Relations,
BMI, Nashville, Tennessee

There is a light...and it is in Janie Lidey's soul. It's in her heart, her words, her melodies and it is contagious to all who come in contact with her. You can't help but feel the love and positive energy when Janie speaks or sings. She is a blessing! Listen and you will agree.

~ Butch Baker ~
Senior Vice President of Creative Services,
HoriPro Entertainment, Nashville, TN

Radiating Hope

Radiating Hope

Cancer Unplugged

Janie Lidey

Foreword by Les Brown

HybridGlobal
PUBLISHING

Published by
Hybrid Global Publishing
301 E 57th Street, 4th fl
New York, NY 10022

Manufactured in the United States of America, or in the United Kingdom when distributed elsewhere.

Lidey, Janie
Radiating Hope: Cancer Unplugged
LCCN: 2018961491
ISBN: 978-1-948181-31-0

Cover design by: Joe Potter / joepotter.com
Copyediting: DJ Montgomery
Interior design: Medlar Publishing Solutions Pvt Ltd., India
Photo credits: Val and Stephanie Westover

www.janielidey.com

I dedicate this book to
all who have loved me back to health.

Contents

Acknowledgements

The things I write about could not come from a heart untouched by God's love and the love of humankind. I wish to express my deep love and appreciation for all who have helped me continue to radiate hope as I have journeyed through an unexpected cancer diagnosis and become a miracle girl in the process.

To God—For Radiating Hope and Love into the core of my being and showering me with Blessings and Miracles.

To Sean and Tristan—For always 'acting as if' I am perfectly healthy and loving me through this journey. I love you to FOREVERVILLE...

To My Team of Doctors: Torrey Smith, Musaberk Goksel, Larry Daugherty, Brian Hougham and John Collins—For combining your expertise with hope and Love, and believing me when I said that *incurable* just doesn't work for me.

To Mum—For always making me feel like I am making a difference in our big, beautiful world.

To my sisters Kris, Sue and Carol and my brother Bill—For always being there for me and believing in my optimism.

To my brother-in-law Dave McHone—For joining the *Radiating Hope* team to summit my prayer flag on Mt. Kilimanjaro. You are a true hero.

To Buzz and Kerry MacPherson—For caring so deeply.

To Reeney O'Reilley—For being with me even when you're not.

To Craig Duswalt—For always making me feel like a Rock Star.

To Skip Franklin—For always believing in my dream.

To DJ Montgomery—For helping me keep my authentic voice alive in your edits.

To Carol Casas—For your special input throughout this project.

To Kevin Tubbs—For always believing I'd be the miracle girl.

To Karen Strauss—For your love and support as my publisher.

To Joe Potter—For your amazing graphics.

To Val and Stef Westover—For always capturing my authenticity in our photo shoots.

To all my extended family, friends and fans… It takes a village and I am so blessed to have you in my life. I'm wishing you all Blessings and Miracles.

And thank you to my special guest authors for your grace and presence:

Dr. John and Tami Collins, Dr. Larry Daugherty, Gene Ehmann, Iklim Goksel, Tom McGuire, David McHone, Dave Nassaney, Dr. Torrey Smith and Matt Wilder.

Foreword by Les Brown

Janie Lidey is a dynamic speaker and creative writer. Her new book, *Radiating Hope,* is designed to transform and inspire millions of people around the world. Janie has always chosen to be a voice of hope even while facing her greatest challenge, cancer. Janie's love, drive and passion for life radiates brighter than ever. Being a twenty-seven year cancer conqueror myself, I have come to learn that it is not what happens to you in life but how you choose to deal with it. It starts with an invincible mindset. The Book of Life says, "As a man thinketh in his heart so is he." *Radiating Hope* gives a clear path to a healthier mind-state, which in turn affects your entire wellbeing.

Are you facing health challenges or looking to improve any area of your life? Janie takes you by the hand and leads you on the path to incorporating the power of love, affirmations, visualization and meditation. She has tried and proven methods that I have used personally, which I know will help to create a healing environment for your life and the lives of others. Janie has been my mentor and she offers you some of her powerful disciplines and lessons to help you strengthen your mind, body and spirit.

This is a fun, easy and spiritual blueprint that will transform your life and change the way you view the world.

You have greatness in you. That's my story and I am sticking to it!

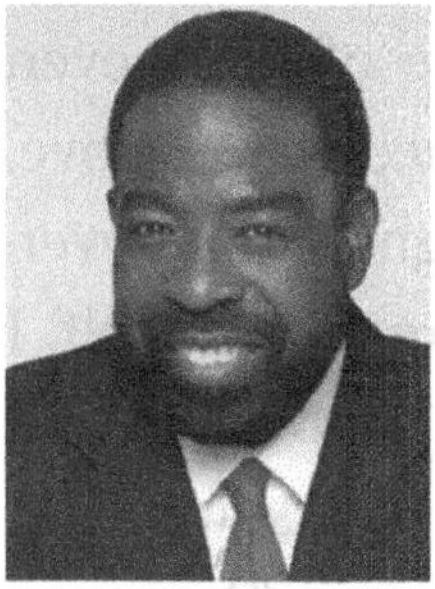

Introduction

It is often in the darkest skies that we see the brightest stars.

~ Richard Evans ~

On a Thursday morning in March of 2018, I was sitting in the audience at Craig Duswalt's Rockstar Marketing Boot Camp in Los Angeles, California when my name was drawn out of a bag of over 500 business cards. I was called to the stage to collect the hundred-dollar bill that Craig was giving away that morning at his event. This might have just been a case of really good luck, but I believe it was more than that. I believe that synchronicity got me on Craig's stage that morning so that I would have the opportunity to share a little piece of the journey I had been on in the months leading up to the event. The hope that I was able to radiate into the audience that morning was part of speaking my miracle into existence.

After Craig gave me my hundred dollar bill, he announced to his audience that I had been diagnosed with stage IV, metastatic breast cancer just a few months earlier and then asked me to share a few words about what I was going through. These are the words that came out of my mouth that morning. "I am the luckiest girl in the world and I believe in blessings and miracles every day. A miracle is a miracle. It doesn't matter if it is stage I or stage IV. The miracle doesn't judge." Just five weeks later, only five months after being diagnosed with what the doctors told me was incurable stage IV metastatic breast cancer, I was cancer free.

Radiating Hope ~ Cancer Unplugged is my vehicle for sharing this story with you. It is a place where I can lift you up and inspire you to believe in blessings and miracles. My prayer for you as you read this book is that the stories and songs will be instrumental in opening your mind, body and spirit to your quiet power within, help you lean into your purpose and see that whatever you are going through in your life, be it cancer or any other life challenge, can be harnessed as a blessing and lead you to *your* miracles.

I have designed this book in a similar format as my first two books, *The Magic of A Song* and *Leap of Faith*

~ *8 Daily Habits to Power Up Your Leap*. In each chapter I will share some of my favorite quotes, an inspirational story from my journey and then at the end of each chapter you will hear from some very special guest authors. They are people whom I have been empowered and inspired by in my life, and I have asked them to share one of their special stories with you. I have included some Daily Action Steps after each guest author's story and finally, each chapter will end with a song. As I have leaned into my gift as a songwriter, I have come to realize the power of music to lift you up, raise your vibration, calm your fear and infuse you with a sense of hope and healing on your journey.

And now, Up, Up & Away...

About the Song "Up, Up & Away"

Marlo Thomas, who starred in a show called *That Girl* when I was growing up, inspired this song. She was always bopping around with such vibrancy and somehow, throughout my life, I have felt like *That Girl*. Marlo serves as National Outreach Director for St. Jude Children's Hospital, which was founded by her father Danny Thomas in 1962.

I am sharing this song with you here in hopes of inspiring you to believe that even when it rains there will always be a rainbow, and maybe you'll be the one to find the pot of gold.

Up, Up & Away

Inspired by Marlo Thomas
Music & Lyrics By Janie Lidey, BMI

A good night's sleep a cup of coffee
The light of day and I'm on my way
A few good thoughts a good song on the radio
And I gotta say

Up up and away my sky has no limit
This is my day
Up up and away my sun is shining
And I'm feeling okay
And I'm expecting miracles
And blessings all along the way
This is my day

Sometimes I stay up too late and get up way too early
But I still jump up ready to rock 'n' roll
And even if it rains I know there'll be a rainbow
And maybe I'll be the one to find the pot o' gold

Up up and away my sky has no limit
This is my day
Up up and away my sun is shining
And I'm feeling okay

And I'm expecting miracles
And blessings all along the way
This is my day

I am a daughter a mom and a wife
A sister a friend and a lover of life
Who knows what else I could be by the end of the day

Up up and away my sky has no limit
This is my day
Up up and away my sun is shining
And I'm feeling okay
And I'm expecting miracles
And blessings all along the way
This is my day
Yeah I'm expecting miracles
And blessings all along the way
This is my day!

CHAPTER #1

Expect Blessings and Miracles

Miracles happen every day. Change your perception of what a miracle is and you'll see them all around you.

~ Jon Bon Jovi ~

What is *your* definition of a blessing or miracle? Perception is everything after all.

On December 1, 2017, I came home from a doctor appointment with a brand new blessing in my life. When I arrived home, my husband Sean was in the garage working on one of his car projects and when he saw the eager look on my face, he put his tools down, pulled up a couple of our comfy shop chairs and invited me to sit down and share my new story with him. On that day, I was given a very special gift. On that day, the miracle I am about to share with you became a possibility. In order for me to help you absorb this miracle in full, I will begin with the events that took place in the years leading up to that day.

In 2011, I took an early retirement from a twenty-six year career as a music educator in Alaska. After teaching native Alaskan kids in some remote, fly-in only villages for three years, a year of classroom music in a couple of elementary schools in Anchorage, five years at a middle school in Eagle River and seventeen years as the choir director and guitar teacher at East Anchorage High School, I realized that it was my time to shift. It was time to leave a job I had done for most of my adult life and start focusing on my journey as a singer-songwriter, author and inspirational speaker. I was ready to motivate on a grander scale. I had attended a convention in Washington D.C. a few years prior to retiring and when I heard the Dalai Lama say, "The women of the west will save the world", every hair rose up on my body and I felt as though the universe was speaking directly to me that I was one of those women. I have been humbly asking the universe ever since that day, "How can I serve?"

When I set out on this journey during what I would consider the mid-afternoon of my life (thinking of you, Wayne Dyer), I did so with the intention that my purpose in life was to raise the vibration of love on our planet through my music and message. I am deeply moved by the thought that we are coming back to Love and that we will be brought back into balance by the power of Love. During my twenty-six years as a teacher, I saw the power Love held in its ability to create positive change in kids' lives. My purpose now is to create that positive change on a global scale.

My husband Sean encouraged me to start my journey with a trip to Nashville where I could network with other songwriters and begin to grow into my new role as singer-songwriter, author and speaker. While in Nashville, I began to honor my new calling by writing my first book and companion CD titled, *The Magic of A Song*. Over the course of the six years that passed leading up to my big miracle, I experienced a myriad of blessings along the way. I woke up each and every day expecting good things to happen and with that expectation in continual motion, good things happened. I had the blessing of co-writing with John Carter Cash, Wesley Orbison and friends. I got to perform at Willie Nelson's 80th birthday tribute in downtown Nashville along with John Carter Cash. I was able to attract the same platinum album musicians to play and sing on my albums that played on the best of the best country recordings in Nashville. I had the opportunity to be interviewed on Craig Duswalt's *Rock Your Life TV* by actor, producer and director Dean Cain, who played Superman in the television hit series and now does a lot of hosting on shows like *The Today Show*. And the list goes on. People kept asking me, "Janie, why are you so lucky? You just seem so blessed." After years of contemplating the answer to that question, I have come to realize that it has nothing to do with luck and everything to do with how I choose to live my life. I expect blessings and miracles every single day. I see because I believe. If you have to see it to believe it, try flipping your perception upside down and see the miracles appear before your very eyes. For some reason, people have got it in their minds that miracles have to be as paramount as Jesus walking on water or Moses parting the Red Sea. But the thing is, miracles happen every single day. Miracles are waiting to unfold for the eye of the believer. The key to seeing miracles begins with believing that you will. The key to being blessed begins with believing that you are.

Six years into my journey as a singer-songwriter, author and inspirational speaker, my career was really taking off. I had successfully launched my best selling *Leap of Faith* book and companion CD and had been doing lots of shows around the country. One of my songs had won the Nashville Songwriters Association International Song Pick. I had been chosen to receive the RockStar Inspiration Award at a big marketing event in LA and I was getting ready to finish off my year performing at Craig Duswalt's *Rock Your Life Night*: a faith-based event at the City National Grove of Anaheim in Southern California. I had co-written the theme song for this event that would be touring globally in the coming years and I was part of the line up. I would be speaking/singing at each event and would be performing with the band singing my newly released song, *Rock Your Life*. I was reaching people in many corners of the world and doing exactly what I had set out to do when I took that leap of faith from my teaching career. My music and message was creating hope and healing in people's lives and I was raising the vibration of Love on our planet. The blessings and miracles were flowing.

The night after this amazing *Rock Your Life* event, I woke up at 2 AM with pain surging from my right hip to my ankle radiating with such intensity, I could barely walk. My leg felt like a tooth in the dentist's chair being drilled on non-stop with no Novocain. I was supposed to get up at 4 AM that morning, take a shower and head up to Los Angeles for a three-day Master Mind event and since I couldn't sleep with all the pain, I decided to just get up and get ready for the drive. I hobbled to the shower, ate some breakfast, filled my to-go coffee cup and headed up the coast highway. I have to say that I am a pretty badass chick with a relatively high pain threshold, but this pain was beyond something I could pretend my way through. I cried my way all the way to LA and upon arrival, I realized that the only choice for me at this point was to drive back to Newport Beach and find a chiropractor. I had been staying with my sister Kris so she set me up with hers and I thought I would just get an adjustment and be back at the Master Mind that afternoon. Instead, I ended up on heavy-duty pain meds and had to cancel all three days. I'm not usually one to take heavy narcotics but when my sister saw the kind of wincing I was doing, she insisted I take the meds. They didn't take the pain away but just took a little bit of the edge off. I flew home to Alaska that week and scheduled an MRI. The story I shared with my husband Sean in the garage on that December afternoon began with the test results that I received from that MRI.

> *It's not what happens to you but how you react that matters.*
>
> ~ Epictetus ~

When I told Sean that I had been diagnosed with stage IV metastatic breast cancer, something inside of him somehow knew how to radiate hope into me. From the very moment he learned of the diagnosis he just looked at me and said, "This is just like a bad cold sweetie. You're gonna be fine. Whatever it is, the medicine will melt it away." He also said that we would have fun with this. We actually sat and talked and laughed and continued dreaming big, as we do no matter what we are going through. We talked about how much I would enjoy getting to know all of the people I would be meeting, how we'd get to spend a ton of time together while he drove me to all of my many appointments, how this would connect me to more people who would benefit from my healing music and message and how this would help me become a more powerful speaker. Maybe the biggest blessing was that this would give me the opportunity to show the world and myself the blessings that appear when we choose Love over fear and the miracles that happen when we choose to live by faith. I had, after all just spent the last two years travelling around the country doing inspirational talks and concerts on the topic of my last book and CD, *Leap of Faith ~ 8 Daily Habits to Power Up Your Leap.* I had been teaching people to expect blessings and miracles in their lives and now I was being faced with one of the greatest opportunities to prove the worth of my daily habits. The miracle that became a possibility back on that December day became a reality on April 27, 2018. Just five short months after being diagnosed with incurable stage IV metastatic breast cancer, my PET scan showed not one single cancer cell lighting up in my body. I am cancer free.

> *Out of difficulties grow miracles.*
>
> ~ Jean de la Bruyere ~

Over the course of the five months leading up to my miracle, I was blessed with a team of doctors that believed in a more holistic approach to my healing. I believe the traditional medical philosophies combined with the holistic mind, body, spirit approach was what led to my quick recovery. Dr. Musaberk Goksel, MD, FACP, was one of those doctors and I have asked him to share a few thoughts with you:

> In medical school, 10th century Persian physician and philosopher Avicenna's teachings influenced me profoundly. Although he was an avid researcher on disease prevention and was preoccupied with finding treatment modalities for ailments, he was also a humanist who reminded doctors of their humanity. In his works, he advises doctors to use their five senses (smell, touch, sight, hearing, and taste) when examining their

patients. This holistic approach in medicine has been a reminder to me every day in my Oncology practice that possibilities, hope, and healing lie within us as long as we stay true to ourselves, learn how to connect with others and embrace both the spiritual and physical aspects of our bodies. It has been very inspiring to observe that Janie Lidey is one of those individuals who knows how to integrate these qualities into her life.

Thank you Dr. Goksel for healing from your heart. I am so blessed that the universe wove you into my life.

And now, I'd like to introduce you to my friend and special guest author, Gene Ehmann. I asked Gene to share his story in this chapter because he too has expected blessings and miracles and has seen the power of God working to bring him back to health.

My Miracle

I had a wonderful, overwhelming encounter with God in the form of a medical miracle, or rather several miracles. These miracles changed everything for my wife Maryann and me, and now, two years later, those miracles continue.

For decades I was a science, evidence, proof guy, and to some extent I still am. Based on those firm beliefs, I studied science, history and bible interpretation before coming to faith. Perhaps the most eye-opening verse for me at the beginning of my walk with the Lord was, *"Now faith is the substance of things hoped for, the evidence of things not seen."* This is ironic on the one hand, and an "of course" occurrence on the other hand, right? Basing my thinking on "evidence", why wouldn't a different take on evidence come before me? How can things "not seen" be evidence? Yet, in my journey coming to faith, I had decided that the Bible is true in its ideas, concepts and words. Now, I've come to understand that there is more "real" in the unseen than in what we see.

At the end of a day in August of 2016, ironically while reading my bible on my phone, the words I was reading seemed jumbled. I thought that the software of the program might be corrupted so I turned off the phone and went to sleep. The next morning I turned on the phone, opened the bible app, and while I had no problem seeing the icons, the words again seemed a bit jumbled. Each time I tried to focus, they didn't make real sense and each time they looked different.

I told Maryann what I was reading and she went to her bible, opened the same verses, and asked me to read. The words came out of my mouth with difficulty, as they didn't quite make sense in the order in which they were presented. I had read those verses dozens of times, yet even when I tried reading them slowly, they made no sense. She told me that what I was reading wasn't what was written. We decided we needed to go to the hospital right away. Maryann drove and when we arrived, she told the ER intake what the problem was and I was quickly admitted. I was seen almost immediately and the ER doctor ordered an MRI. I barely recall having the test and shortly after, the ER doc came out and said very, very hesitatingly, "You have something in your brain that doesn't belong there."

We asked if we could see the image and the doc rolled out the CRT-like machine so we could see the results. There was a large tumor pressing on the area of the brain that affected my reading and the diagnosis was Metastatic Melanoma. The doc was very affected by this, seemingly even more so than we were. In fact, Maryann and I felt no panic or fear. We asked the doc who we should see next and after looking around as if to make sure no one was listening, he softly said that he would go to Barrows in St. Joseph's hospital. We got the impression that he wasn't supposed to send us somewhere else.

We had to get an ambulance to St Joseph's and en route Maryann called our daughter Rebecca and told her what was going on. Rebecca said that a young man in her church had recently had very successful brain surgery performed at Barrows. The surgeon's name was Porter, and she believed that he too was a believer, so we might look for him.

We arrived at St. Joseph's and as soon as they heard the issue, they informed us that the doctor on duty for brain issues was Dr. Randall Porter! Wow! My memory is we met with him very quickly. In fact, we had arrived at the hospital on Saturday and we saw Dr. Porter on Sunday. We told him of our referral to him, reminded him of his work with the young man at our daughter's church, and he remembered that. We said we heard he was a believer, which he confirmed, and when we asked if we could pray together, he readily agreed. He said the surgery was pretty straightforward from what he could see, and that it would take anywhere from two to four hours. I was scheduled for the surgery the very next day.

Early morning Monday, as we were rolling into the OR, we again prayed with Dr. Porter. About an hour later, I was in recovery. The doctor came into my room and said that the surgery had taken 48 minutes from open to close!!! His attending surgeon was standing with him and Dr. Porter said that when he opened my skull, the tumor popped out! It had not been attached to my brain tissue. His attending made a cork popping sound and confirmed what Dr. Porter said. A miracle!

We were delighted, of course. As I was "coming to" the verse came to me, Psalm 118:17, "You shall not die, but live, and declare the works of the Lord." The news of the surgery and that verse put me in a state of euphoria, which lasted for weeks and weeks. The doctor cleared me to go home the next day, and but for a mix up on meds by the discharge physician, I would have. Nevertheless, I was home in four days.

From that time forward, I have felt and lived the Love of God. Maryann performed the work of an angel as she took care of me in the weeks that followed. I felt no pain or discomfort at all as she devoted herself to seeing me get rest and recovery.

Several weeks after surgery, I had a gamma knife radiation treatment, which was followed by a brain hemorrhage that required a second surgery. But with the wonderful care and love from the Lord, my wife and our family, I had no pain or discomfort. After the second surgery, I had to have immunotherapy and with that came multiple side effects and discomfort. Still, my lovely wife continued loving and serving me.

I'd never want anyone to go through what I have. That said, it has been one of the best events in my life *feeling* the Lord, hearing from Him and having an angel touch my head as a physical reassurance that, indeed, God is with me. He loves me! Today, I am clear! Maryann and I continue to expect miracles and like Janie said earlier, “the key to seeing miracles begins with believing that you will. The key to being blessed begins with believing that you are.”

What a wonderful life!

Daily Action Steps

- Sit quietly and just breathe. Acknowledge your quiet power within and allow that power to create healing in you.

- Think about a blessing in your life. Write down a blessing you would like to see happen in your future, and then sit quietly and feel how you would feel if that blessing already existed. Remember, the key to being blessed begins with believing that you are.

- Imagine a miracle that you would like to see happen in your life. Allow yourself to believe that your miracle already exists and that all you must do to see it is believe that it will unfold for you. And when in doubt, just keep believing. Remember, the key to seeing miracles begins with believing that you will.

About the Song "Abundance"

This song came to life at a faith-based event in Coronado Bay, California. Maryann Ehmann invited me to sing and speak at her annual event called, *Create Your Magnificent Year*, and while there, one of the attendees, my good friend Cindy Baldwin, reached over and handed me a few lines of a poem she had written that morning. I took those words, added a few of my own thoughts and then created this song for the final morning of our seminar.

I am sharing this song with you here in hopes of inspiring you to create your day rather than your day creating you. It is in the here and now that we use our power to create our own reality by stepping out in faith and expecting Blessings and Miracles.

Abundance

Inspired by Cindy Baldwin,
Maryann Ehmann and Nick Castellano
Music by Janie Lidey, BMI
Lyrics by Cindy Baldwin & Janie Lidey

Abundance does grow on trees
It runs in the grass and it swims in the seas
It is the ocean the sun and the breeze
Abundance does grow on trees

Create you day rather than your day creating you
Abundance does grow on trees
Blessings and Miracles every single day
Abundance does grow on trees

We create our own reality
We can be a mighty oak
If that is what we're called to be
We are Royal we are Epic beyond our wildest dreams
Abundance does grow on trees...

It's in the now we have the power
Every minute of every hour
Our power is lined up with what we're called to do
It's in the now we have the power

Create you day rather than your day creating you
Abundance does grow on trees
Blessings and Miracles every single day
Abundance does grow on trees

We create our own reality
We can be a mighty oak
If that is what we're called to be
We are Royal we are Epic beyond our wildest dreams
Abundance does grow on trees...
Abundance does grow on trees...
Abundance does grow on trees...

CHAPTER #2

Radiate Hope

Hope is being able to see that there is light despite all of the darkness.

~ Desmond Tutu ~

With any medical diagnosis comes the challenge of making choices. And the question is, will we base our choices on our fears or on our hopes? What are you basing your choices on?

On December 3, 2017, just two days after the December 1st stage IV metastatic breast cancer diagnosis, it just so happened that the only Super Moon of 2017 lit up the sky. It is said that there are special healing powers in the super moon and somehow, my husband Sean intuitively tapped into them on that magical night. We had gone up to bed in the loft of our log home on the Anchorage hillside, and the moon was shining so brightly on our bed that it was like laying in the sun. It was radiating light with such intensity that it gave my husband an idea that ended up radiating hope into the very core of our beings. Sean suddenly got this look in his eyes and he told me to take off my clothes and lay in the moonlight (It's not what you're thinking). He said he'd be right back and when he returned from his shop he had a large magnifying glass in his hands. He had taken the smooth, round glass out of its plastic holder and began to place it over my right hip where the doctors said the largest tumor was growing. You know how you can burn a hole through a leaf when you hold a magnifier over it and allow the sun to beam through it? Well Sean's thought was that we could harness the power of the Super Moon by allowing its light to reflect through the glass into my body. He proceeded to let the moonlight shine through the glass and begin to melt away the tumor. He let the smooth glass glide over the parts of my body that were apparently infected and we imagined those unhealthy cells just disappearing. Interestingly, just a few weeks later, a very large growth on the outside of my body that I was supposed to have removed and biopsied that week but had to cancel due to my new diagnosis and scheduled surgery, simply dried up and fell off of my body. I know that God gave us that visual to help us understand the ease with which the growths on the inside of my body would also just melt away. Talk about radiating hope!

One of the first doctors I was scheduled to see after my diagnosis was an orthopedic surgeon. After examining my MRI and then doing some additional follow up x-rays, Dr. Hougham told me that he wasn't going to allow me to walk out of his office without crutches. Apparently the large lesion in my hip area had eaten away so much of my bone that I was literally about to fall over. He was amazed that I was still walking after everything I told him I had been up to during the months leading up to this: Performing concerts around the country and carrying my own heavy gear. Leading Segway Tours around Lake Hood in Alaska. Riding 4-wheelers at our remote cabin. Taking my dog on long summer hikes. Riding bikes. Climbing stairs. Painting from the perch of a tall ladder. It was a miracle that my leg hadn't completely fractured already. And thank God it hadn't, because he said that if it had, this would have been very challenging to fix. In fact, I learned recently that one of my old high school friends had the same thing happen in his hip, but it did fracture and he never walked again.

I am amazed that my intuition actually kept me from doing some of the things that truly could have left me broken. I had declined an offer to go horseback riding while doing a show in Austin, Texas which is crazy considering I grew up with horses and hadn't gotten to ride in a long time. Something inside of me just knew. I had declined an offer to ride the awesome motorcycle my husband got for me even though I would normally have jumped right on. Something inside of me just knew. While everyone else was jumping off the front of the stage at the City National Grove in Anaheim after a photo shoot on the night of the *Rock Your Life* concert, I stood up and took the safe way off. Something inside of me just knew. Thank goodness for intuition.

> *The soul always knows what to do to heal itself. The challenge is to silence the mind.*
>
> ~ Caroline Myss ~

So I left the doctor's office that day on a set of crutches with surgery scheduled for the following week. There was a biopsy the next day and that was followed by the implant of a titanium rod placed through my right femur and attached with screws at the hip and knee. There was really no choice on this decision. I had to stabilize the bone in my leg and this was the only way. It's kind of funny that when I was growing up, one of my favorite TV shows was *The Bionic Woman*. I loved how

Jamie Summers used the strength she gained from her many surgeries to create good in the world. So many people told me over the years that I reminded them of Lindsay Wagner, who played Jamie Summers in the show, and now I was getting to become the Bionic Woman.

A healer's power stems not from any special ability, but from maintaining the courage and awareness to embody and express the universal healing power that every human being naturally possesses.
~ Eric Michaël Leventhal ~

After the surgery, I would have to choose whether or not to have radiation. My team of doctors recommended this as part of my treatment plan so I decided to go with it. My intuition had done a pretty good job for me so far and my gut was telling me that I should follow their advice on this. I really liked my radiation oncologist, Dr. Larry Daugherty and I felt safe saying yes to his recommendation of just ten short sessions of radiation. Larry seemed to radiate hope into me with his loving presence and with that blessing, I just knew that miracles would follow.

Shortly after saying yes to doing radiation, my dear friend and author, Suzy Prudden called to invite me to be a part of the 'word' book she was writing. She suggested to me that my word should be *Radiate.* She said, "You radiate Love in everything you do Janie." I loved that thought and it helped me take a different look at the radiation process. I decided to put my imagination to work and during each radiation session, I lay on the table and rather than see something burning into my body to kill something bad, I chose to see love radiate into my body and allow those unhealthy cells to just melt away. I remember thinking about how important it is to love without condition and I applied that to my procedure. I loved those cancer cells right out of my body. I thanked them for coming to awaken me and lead me deeper into my purpose and then I invited them to make their exit. I thought about the students I used to teach and how some of them were very toxic but when I infused them with love, those toxicities tended to disappear and their true, healthy self came to life. I simply loved those toxic cells for the lessons they brought me and then lovingly allowed the radiation to help melt them right out of my body.

> *An awakened imagination works with a purpose. It creates and conserves the desirable, and transforms or destroys the undesirable.*
>
> ~ Neville Goddard ~

On the last day of my radiation treatments, the staff at the Alaska Cancer Treatment Center had a celebration waiting for me in the lobby. They gave me a beautiful basket filled with healthy goodies, had me ring the special gong they have all their patients ring upon completion of treatment and then presented me with a prayer flag that would be carried to the top of Mt. Kilimanjaro as part of the tradition my radiation oncologist Dr. Larry Daugherty had established through his *Radiating Hope* Foundation.

And now, I'd like to introduce you to Dr. Larry Daugherty. I chose Larry to be one of my special guest authors for this chapter because he is the founder of *Radiating Hope* and has a special story to tell.

Climbing for a Cure

Habiba. Her name means "one who is loved." Yet here she lies, alone and afraid in a hospital bed in Moshi, Tanzania. Suspicion and superstition is strong among her family regarding her cervical cancer diagnosis. In their tribal language, the word "cancer" does not even really exist. To them, she is cursed. And so Habiba is here now. Alone. And Afraid. Dying. Dying of cancer. Dying from cancer. One that could be cured. One that should be cured.

Cured? Yes. The cure for cancer does exist for millions upon millions of people all around the world. Modern technology has exploded with respect to targeted and precise treatments that can literally cure the majority of cancers when caught at an early stage. Habiba's cancer is not early stage. Despite this, her cervical cancer very likely could be treated successfully and curatively for the Tanzanian equivalent of about $300 US dollars.

As a radiation oncologist and visitor to Tanzania, I am horrified to learn of the complete lack of cancer care in Moshi, Tanzania. There quite literally, are no local options for Habiba. No access to a chemotherapy infusion center whatsoever. No lifesaving radiation services for one of the most radiosensitive diseases in the spectrum of oncology. In a country of over fifty-five million people, I learn that Tanzania has only one working radiation machine and this machine is decades old and often nonfunctional. By U.S. standards, this country needs hundreds more of these expensive and complex machines to fulfill even basic oncology needs. So today, I come to emotional grips that Habiba will die. It is so unfair. So tragic. I meet many more Habibas during my subsequent tours of the Kilimanjaro Christian Medical Center in Tanzania. And the Kathmandu Cancer Center in

Nepal. And center after center in developing countries around the globe.

Within our collective reach is the ability to literally extend blessings and miracles to millions upon millions of people who face a cancer diagnosis without any access to treatment. It is for this purpose that *Radiating Hope* was imagined. To improve access to cancer care around the globe. The challenges are enormous and, at times, daunting. Hurdles include lack of education, cancer screening, appropriate training, inadequate electrical grids and lack of resources to pay for radiation machines that can cost millions of dollars each.

The humble roots of *Radiating Hope* began to sprout in the unlikeliest of places. Any other seed perhaps would not have germinated in the harsh winter environment of New Hampshire's Mt. Washington. In 1934, a gust reaching 231 miles per hour would set the new world record for wind speed at the summit of this peak. While among the tallest mountains east of the Mississippi, standing at 6,288 feet of elevation, this peak is nearly insignificant in comparison to the giants of the Himalayas. However, at its wintry summit in 2010, two oncology-bound residents and mountaineers unfurled a strand of Tibetan prayer flags and boldly proclaimed their mission to improve the state of cancer care around the globe. As the flags flapped in the mounting storm, threads broke free into the wind, carrying their prayer to the heavens. This is the day *Radiating Hope* was born.

Since that day, thousands of prayer flags have been carried to the summits of the highest mountains around the globe on behalf of those afflicted with cancer. Flags become threads and threads become prayers as teams of climbers raise money to provide oncology services to regions of the world where this is nonexistent.

When asked why he would attempt to climb Mt. Everest, George Mallory's now immortal response was, "Because it is there." When asked why *we* climb mountains, our response typically is, "Because it is not there." Cancer treatment unfortunately is nonexistent in most of the regions of the world where our organization encourages lay mountaineers, cancer patients and oncologists to ascend to the top of the highest summits. Prayer flags in their backpacks, climbers dedicate their journey to loved ones, friends or patients afflicted by cancer. Funds are raised and in this way a cure is passed along, a miracle extended, to a Habiba in Tanzania or to a Sherpa in a remote mountain village in Nepal.

As an oncologist, climbing with colleagues and patients has given me an enormous measure of empathy for the cancer journey. In the mountains, I took Zofran for the first time to palliate my own nausea from altitude sickness. In the mountains, I have experienced headaches, fatigue, gastrointestinal distress and many of the symptoms that my patients experience during their own treatment.

I always feel I return from the mountains a better doctor. When I met Janie Lidey in 2017, I was recovering from the physical and emotional toll of my unsuccessful bid to climb Mt Everest. My team had to turn around just 98 excruciatingly small meters from the summit due to high winds. It is perhaps impossible to convey the disappointment I felt at having come so close to fulfilling a lifelong dream. However, meeting Janie snapped me out of my funk. Full of life, full of love, full of faith and so very unfairly, Janie was diagnosed with metastatic breast cancer at seemingly the pinnacle of her own life. Several months after meeting Janie, on a day when I learned that my oncology mentor and hero, Luther Brady had died, she arrived at my clinic, guitar in hand and cheered my heart and spirit with her newly written song, *Radiating Hope.* Janie had no idea what I was going through that day but after playing the song she had written for this chapter and then learning of Luther's passing that very day, she decided to dedicate the song in loving memory of Luther Brady. Janie has restored my belief in miracles.

And now I'd like to introduce you to my brother-in-law David McHone. I asked Dave to be one of my special guest authors here because when he learned that my prayer flags would be carried to the top of Mt. Kilimanjaro, he was determined to be the one to summit my flags.

Bucket List With a Purpose

On January 25, 2018, I received some news from my sister-in-law Janie Lidey that changed the trajectory of my year. Janie had been diagnosed with stage IV metastatic breast cancer in December of 2017, and after completing her radiation treatments in January, she was given a set of prayer flags that would be carried to the top of Mt. Kilimanjaro as part of a ceremonial healing tradition created by a foundation called *Radiating Hope.* When I got wind of her news, I asked if I could be the one to summit Janie's flags. Climbing Mt. Kilimanjaro had been on my bucket list for years and as soon as I heard about the climb, I knew that I was meant to carry Janie's flags to the top of the mountain.

Janie's mindset was already working to make her a survivor but it takes a village and in my infinite wisdom, I thought I would help her live to a great old age by summiting her prayer flags. So in February of 2018, I signed up with the *Radiating Hope* team and began my journey to not only be instrumental in Janie's healing, but also to help create hope and healing for cancer patients in remote areas of the world. I was able to raise over five thousand dollars for Radiating Hope, climb with a Rockstar team and ultimately, summit Janie's flags while checking a life long dream off of my bucket list.

Mt. Kilimanjaro is the tallest and most recognizable mountain in Africa and takes climbers through five different eco-systems to its summit at 19,341 feet. Reaching the peak of a mountain of this caliber has really changed my understanding of the world. I did the climb out of a desire to make a difference in Janie's life and the lives of those in less fortunate countries and in the end, the climb made me realize how much I meant to the people in my own life.

I started training for this amazing adventure at the age of 66. I had not done a lot of research on the climb, as I didn't care about the dangers and the obstacles ahead. I just knew I was going to summit with Janie's flags. Climbing relies on self-management, mental strength and determination to reach one's goals, however, events can go terribly wrong. On the first day of the journey, I forged ahead through a rainy climate with only one climber able to keep pace. On the second day we split into two groups and I climbed with the faster group. On day three, I slowed down and spent time looking at flowers and the incredible views that I had missed when all I was doing was looking at my boots and climbing as fast as I could the first two days. By day four, things took a turn for the worse for me. The Diamox (high altitude sickness medicine) I was taking made me lose my appetite completely and I became severely dehydrated. I had to mix carbs with sugar and milk to get strength for the summit. I could not even look at any food but forced it down knowing that if I wanted to leave for the summit at 11:45 pm on the final leg of the climb, I had to hold down some food. I was now on my own as far as mental strength and determination to reach the summit, but I was assigned a private coach to keep me safe and make sure I drank enough water. He had no idea what he signed up for. He kept saying *pole pole* for *slow slow*. I had one focus and determination and that was to keep going. If I stopped I might have frozen there and not summited. My mind was now on autopilot and I just kept putting one foot in front of the other. My coach tried to stop me at the first summit posts but my idea of summiting was to keep going until there was no higher land within eyesight. I had carried many flags for Janie to the summit but I also had four special flags that all of my sponsors had signed to support Radiating Hope, Janie, and my climb, and I was determined to summit them all.

Ascending and descending a mountain like Kilimanjaro can bring about emotions not unlike those that a cancer patient might go through. There is the hope of reaching the top and the hope of becoming cancer free. There is the pain that the body feels as it is breaking down from the intensity of the climb and the pain of going through the diagnosis, treatment and healing from cancer. I experienced a myriad of setbacks on my journey but ultimately I survived. I had a severe case of dehydration on the ascent, suffered a hyperextended knee on the descent and after traveling home on four different airlines with pain so excruciating I felt like I could die, I was whisked off to the emergency room and diagnosed with acute pancreatitis.

It took a few months to recover from the climb, but all is well now. I am so grateful to the *Radiating Hope* team and my sponsors for the opportunity to take part in this journey. I am grateful that my sister-in law Janie is now cancer free. And I am grateful to be working on my next bucket list wish.

Daily Action Steps

- Sit quietly and think about the word Radiate. What kind of glow do you emit from within that you can light up the world with? What can you do today to Radiate Hope?

- Think about someone you know who seems to be in a bit of a dark place in his or her life. How might you be a beacon of light for them today?

- As you go through your day today, stop to radiate love and hope to a part of your body that needs some healing. Send some big love to your cells.

About the Song "Radiating Hope"

This song came to life after learning about the *Radiating Hope* Foundation that my radiation oncologist created to help bring medical technologies to less fortunate places in the world. When I found out that the prayer flag I was presented with after completing radiation would be carried to the top of Mt. Kilimanjaro, and that my brother in law Dave McHone wanted to be the one to summit my flag, this song came pouring out of me.

I am sharing this song with you here in hopes of inspiring you to believe in your power to be a radiant light creating hope for a better tomorrow.

Radiating Hope

Inspired by Larry Daugherty and Dave McHone
Dedicated to the memory of Luther Brady
Music by Janie Lidey, BMI & Matt Wilder, ASCAP
Lyrics by Janie Lidey, BMI

We're living in a time an awakening in in life
Where people wanna shine a brighter light
There's so much to give to ease the sorrow
Radiating hope for a better tomorrow

Radiating Hope Radiating Life
Radiating Warmth Radiating Light
Radiating Love Radiating Faith
Coming out of the dark to light a better way

There's a feeling in the air
There are blessings everywhere
And people wanna show how much they care
There are mountains to be climbed
We can lead or we can follow
Radiating hope for a better tomorrow

Radiating Hope Radiating Life
Radiating Warmth Radiating Light
Radiating Love Radiating Faith
Coming out of the dark to light a better way

Where there is fear there is love
You get to choose what you're made of
When you choose love you avoid the fight
And you radiate with light

Radiating Hope Radiating Life
Radiating Warmth Radiating Light
Radiating Love Radiating Faith
Radiating Hope Radiating Life
Radiating Warmth Radiating Light
Radiating Love Radiating Faith
Coming out of the dark to light a better way
Coming out of the dark to light a better way
Coming out of the dark to light a better way

CHAPTER #3

Fly High

Capture your dreams and your life becomes full. You can, because you think you can.

~ Nikita Koloff ~

One of the most vivid dreams I have during my sleeping hours is one I have dreamt over and over again. I started having this dream when I was a little girl, and when I am in it I know that my only requirement for succeeding is that I must believe with all of my might that I can fly. I am simply standing on the ground and with complete faith and one giant leap I begin to soar. There is no fear in my dream (in fact I know that if I allow even the slightest amount of fear to creep in, I will not be successful), and I know that all I must truly do is act as if I can fly, and I do. My flying dream has taught me that I can do anything I imagine. As long as

I calm my fear, act as if, and leap with faith, I end up flyin' high! What are you dreaming about in your life and what are you doing to allow yourself to fly high?

As far back as I remember having my flying dreams, I also remember having daydreams about spreading peace and love across our planet. I know, it sounds kinda corny, but at twelve years of age, I had a sense that this was my purpose on earth. I became a singer-songwriter in the sixth grade, and when I began to play my songs for people, I realized that music would be my vehicle for creating the change I wanted to see in the world. The music I wrote seemed to lift people up, encourage kindness, and bring a sense of calm and even healing to them. I remember thinking, *What if my music could help spread that peace and love across the land?*

Be the change you wish to see in the world.

~ Ghandi ~

While songwriting was my deepest passion and created an amazing path for me, I was also being called to become a teacher. When I went to college, I majored in music education. Upon graduation I was given the most incredible opportunity, not only to teach our youth, but also to live a life that would fuel the writing

I would continue to do through the years. My first job offer was in Seattle, but I decided to accept an offer that required me to calm my fear, act as if, and leap with faith. The job was in a remote, fly-in-only village called Kwigillingok, Alaska!

> *Two roads diverged in a wood and I—I took the one less traveled by, and that has made all the difference.*
>
> ~ Robert Frost ~

The road to Alaska was my road less traveled. Just a few weeks after my December graduation, I boarded a plane in sunny San Francisco, flew to Seattle, changed planes, and headed for Anchorage. There I boarded a smaller plane from Anchorage to Bethel, where I changed planes again and boarded a little Cessna that took me out to the village of Kwigillingok (a.k.a. Kwig) Alaska. I hopped off the Cessna onto a dogsled pulled by a snow machine and was whisked off to my village housing on the banks of the Kuskokwim River. The temperature was nearly 100 degrees colder in Kwig than it was just hours earlier when I left San Francisco! There were only a few hours of daylight at that time of year in Alaska, and what might have been a cozy drive to school in a heated car had I taken the job in

Seattle was instead a ride in the dark from one end of the village to the other on my snow machine in 20 degrees below zero. There was no running water in Kwig, so my bathroom consisted of a honey bucket for a toilet and a cold, wet cloth for bathing each day. My adventures in Kwig were the beginning of a journey that would shape me into the writer and leader I would become.

After traveling as an itinerant music teacher in the villages for three years, I moved to Anchorage, where I spent the remainder of my teaching career. I was excited about the positive change I was making in my school setting, but that big dream I had as a kid kept coming back to me. That childhood dream of spreading peace and love across the planet made me want to shift out of teaching in one building and make the whole world my classroom. So like I said in Chapter One, I decided to take an early retirement from teaching. I decided to calm my fear, act as if and leap with faith. I immersed myself in writing so that I could get back to the dream of using my music to create the positive change I wanted to see in the world.

Seventeen years of teaching in the most diverse high school in the nation taught me so much about what really matters in life. The lessons I learned are the lessons I share in my *Leap of Faith* book. They are also the foundation for the message I share on the stages I now speak and sing from: Act as If, Begin it Now, Dream Big, Just Imagine, Live in Gratitude, Let the Music Lift You, Laugh While You're Cryin' and Leap With Love. I know that my success in life has come from applying these principles in every present moment. I believe it is why I was invited to co-write songs in Nashville with John Carter Cash and friends and sing at Willie Nelson's 80th birthday tribute. I believe it is why I have platinum album musicians playing on my albums. I believe it is why I am being invited to share my message on stages all over the country. I believe it is why people are sharing their stories with me about how my music and message is lifting them up and changing their lives. And I believe it is why I am cancer free just five short months into what was apparently an incurable stage IV metastatic breast cancer diagnosis.

I know that we all have a gift to share with the world. My gift shines brightest when I share my message through my music. It is my deepest desire to inspire you to lean into your gift and use it to create positive change on our beautiful planet. And just remember, as long as you calm your fear, act as if, and leap with faith, you'll end up flyin' high!

Use what talents you possess. The woods would be very silent if no birds sang there except those that sang best.

~ William Blake ~

And now I'd like to introduce you to my new friend and Qigong instructor, Tom McGuire. I asked Tom to share his story here because he is a master at *flyin' high* by transmitting positive energy for others to receive.

The Last Eight Minutes

What if you could take a dreadful situation and turn it around to be a real win! Your challenge seems impossible, then someone comes into your life and shows you how to transform it in a matter of EIGHT minutes.

It was the fall of 1970, a cool night in Omaha, Nebraska's football stadium. The stands were packed with excited fans! I was a defensive back and leader for the University of Northern Colorado's football team. We were losing. The momentum of the game was in Omaha's favor. We were behind 19-0 with EIGHT minutes left! The outcome seemed dreadful.

Coach called the defense together and presented a solution with the belief and intensity that only he could convey. "We have to get a turn-over! Without this we will run out of time! Can you do this?"

Imagine twenty-one points in EIGHT minutes! We looked at each other and said, "Done deal; it's going happen!" We believed, without any doubt, that we could change the outcome. Our distress was transformed to determination instantaneously! The next time out, we intercepted the ball, and the offense gained possession and scored! It seemed like magic as we turned the momentum of the game our way! The Intensity and Belief were contagious!

The opponent just couldn't stop our offense. We were so focused that all doubt vanished. Within minutes we began dominating the game. The final scoreboard read 00:29 seconds, the score 19-22. We won that game! The outcome had been imagined and achieved in EIGHT minutes! Coach showed us that cold night how to turn a dreadful situation into a real win! He used to say, "Football is a Metaphor for Life. When you're down, you have got to get the ball back!"

Fast-forward thirty-five years. I was commissioned to travel to Greeley, Colorado, for a work assignment. It was a cold, winter day, when I arrived in that town. I called Coach for lunch. After all the years that had passed, he sat there talking to me as if we had just finished practice. He was my hero, still coaching and teaching, and now suffering with a deadly cancer.

His inspiration that day was as thrilling and compelling as that cold night in Omaha. He explained: "There are times in life when people are scared, frightened. That's when God calls and sends brave people to inspire them. That's why you're here. Everyone runs out of time. The final EIGHT minutes in life comes for everyone; it's how you play the game that counts. Did you run as fast as you could? Did you do your best? What do you see when you look in the mirror?" Then he looked at me with a squint in his eye, tilting his head and repeated, "That's why you're here, Tommy. That's why you're here."

Coach ran out of time, had his final play on earth. Certainly the Lord has him in a special place. He's in heaven coaching someone how to run backwards or catch a punt. He used to say: "Keep your head in the game. Find that something inside yourself that you never knew you had; then play with all your heart until that final whistle blows!"

During those years, coach made all the difference in my life. He pushed me to the limit, enabling me to find myself. I can hear his voice like it was yesterday, "When you get your ass kicked you better get up. The clock is ticking. You only have so much time; then that final whistle is going to blow, and you damn well better be proud of yourself."

Fast-forward another ten years. Retired, I'm coaching and teaching Qigong classes at the health club. There are two senior men in my class, both using canes to aid their stability. After training and practicing Qigong for two months, they developed enough balance and strength to walk without their canes.

The practice of Qigong is the art of not only cultivating and balancing the energy in myself, but as an instructor, transmitting positive energy for others to receive. Although there has yet to be conclusive evidence that Qigong can cure cancer, it has been medically proven to be an adjunct to cancer treatment. Qigong improves fatigue, immune function, cortisol levels and quality of life. What if it were possible to strengthen someone's immune system with positive energy, helping them to heal?

One morning, an oncologist shared with me a report about the effects of Qigong and how it improves the quality of life for cancer patients. He invited me to teach Qigong at the Cancer Treatment Center.

While teaching Qigong class, I continued to meet committed people battling different types of cancer at different stages. It was December 2017 when a woman named Janie joined my class. She had been diagnosed with Stage IV Metastatic Breast Cancer. She was also told that it was incurable, that it had spread to her hip and sacrum and a tumor was eating away the bone in her leg.

Coach's words echoed in my mind: "Eight minutes left; keep your head in the game. Put your heart into this." Now I understood what Coach said. "That's why you're here." His energy was alive and present. The score was not in Janie's favor. The challenge seemed dreadful, but she believed that she could reverse the outcome. Her Intensity and Belief were contagious! Her presence was saying: "Done deal, this disease is gone!"

The energy of Qi has yet to be accurately measured. How would you measure the Qi that night in Omaha? How do you measure inspiration, hope, or love? How do you measure determination? Someone or something inspires you, then you find something inside of yourself that you never thought was there. The energy of all the years, all the coaching, all the trials, the failures and successes culminate into a desire that cannot stop you. Then you persist with all your heart until that last whistle blows! On April 27, 2018, after four months in cancer treatment and participation in Qigong class, Janie had a PET scan that showed her completely free of cancer. Not one cancer cell in her body!

Voice of Destiny

Listening for your voice
You whisper sparingly
Between words...
Breath of Destiny,
I'm hungry for purpose;
Once again; the road is forked...
Men walk tall in quest of fame
Talk fast yet stay so wayward.
The spring of life has passed,
Sanity; such a high price!
Laughing, loving,
Smiling is easier now...
Echoes and reflections
No longer so sparse!
Listening in silence
For your faithful whisper;
Oh voice of destiny.

~ Tommy ~

Daily Action Steps

- During those quiet moments while lying in bed at night, getting ready to drift off into dreamland, imagine yourself flyin' high in whatever direction you want to fly toward. Who knows what kind of dream you might ignite?

- Find a local Qigong class and give it a try.

- Look over your life's journey and be aware of your gifts and how you shine your brightest light. Commit to lighting up the world each day with your gift.

About the Song "It's Your Time to Fly"

My nephew Scott Casas was about to graduate from college when this song came to life. It is all about being the mighty oak that you are, shining your brightest light and flyin' high.

I am sharing this song with you here in hopes of inspiring you to believe in your power to soar across the sky, spread your mighty wings and fly high.

It's Your Time to Fly

Inspired by Scott Casas

Music & Lyrics by Janie Lidey, BMI

You are a mighty oak grown up from a tiny seed
You are everything that you were meant to be
You are a mighty bird you can soar across the sky
And it's your time to fly

I hope you live every moment one moment at a time
Always reaching higher rising up to meet the sky
In good times and bad times
God will keep you in His sight
Livin' every moment one moment at a time

I'll make a wish for you that you will be strong
And that you'll take the risk
When your passion comes along
That you'll find everlasting love and life will be kind
And you will do the things
You've imagined in your mind

I hope you live every moment one moment at a time
Always reaching higher rising up to meet the sky

In good times and bad times
God will keep you in His sight
Livin' every moment one moment at a time

You are a shining star
And it's not what but who you are
Your light is shining bright and it's your time to fly

I hope you live every moment one moment at a time
Always reaching higher rising up to meet the sky
In good times and bad times
God will keep you in His sight
Livin' every moment one moment at a time

You are a mighty oak grown up from a tiny seed
You are everything that you were meant to be
You are a mighty bird you can soar across the sky
And it's your time to fly

CHAPTER #4

Be Present

The secret of health for both mind and body is not to mourn for the past, worry about the future, or anticipate troubles, but to live in the present moment wisely and earnestly.

~ Buddha ~

One of the questions I have been asked during this healing journey is, "Janie, how do you stay so positive?" My answer to that is simple: "I live in the present." One of the greatest gifts we have is our ability to choose our thoughts. We can choose to live in the past, the future or the present. How are you choosing to live your life?

If we choose to live in the past, we concoct all kinds of stories that can lead us to anger, regret, fear and many other negative feelings. On the day I was diagnosed with cancer, I could have created quite a story for myself based on the past that would have led me to staying sick rather than being well. I could have gone to the thought that if only they would have diagnosed this several years ago this cancer may not have metastasized. Or, if only they had properly diagnosed this when I went to the ER the prior year with so much pain in my back that I couldn't walk then maybe I wouldn't have a titanium rod in my leg. Or, if only the mammograms I have had every single year had detected the lump in my breast, I wouldn't have ended up with a stage IV diagnoses. What good would any of this bring to my healing?

If we choose to live in the future, we concoct all kinds of stories that lead us to worry, anxiety, fear and many other negative feelings. I could have created quite a story for myself based on the future that also would have led me to staying sick rather than being well. I could have worried that now I may not get to see my son graduate from college. I could have wondered if I would ever get to see my son marry. I could have feared that I would not have the chance to make a difference with the music and message I have been developing. What good would any of this bring to my healing?

It is through gratitude for the present moment that the spiritual dimension of life opens up.

~ Eckhart Tolle ~

When we choose to live in the present, our story unfolds in a way that empowers us to live our best life, right here, right now. Once again, I go to my 8 Daily Habits in *Leap of Faith*. I have never actually considered myself living with cancer. When my eyeballs pop open in the morning, I go right to acting as if I am cancer free. I begin thinking about my purpose and how I can be of service. I dream big about the talks I will develop, the songs I will write and the stages I will share those messages from to create hope and healing for millions of people. I imagine my body in perfect health and see my cells rejuvenating through the Love I am sending to them. I get up expecting to feel great and if I feel a little puny from the side effects of the meds I'm on or have pain in my leg from my titanium rod implant, I just imagine feeling magnificent and see myself having an epic day. I go right to gratitude for the opportunities this diagnosis has brought to me. I am grateful for how I have the ability to grow and become more awakened to my purpose and for all God is preparing me for as a speaker, author and singer-songwriter through this experience. I listen to music while meditating, doing chores and driving. I remember to laugh while I'm crying. And finally, I leap with Love. I choose Love over fear. I choose Love when in doubt. I choose Love in every present moment.

Look to this day for it is life. For yesterday is already a dream and tomorrow is only a vision. But today well-lived makes every yesterday a dream of happiness, and every tomorrow a vision of hope.

~ Sanskrit Proverb ~

And now I'd like to introduce you to my dear friend Iklim Goksel. When she and I met, it was as though our spirits had been joined before. I am sharing Iklim's story in this chapter because of the lovely and artistic way she paints a picture of living and loving in the present.

Digging Deep into the Earth

I kneel down on the ground. I am on my knees with excruciating pain but I don't waste my time thinking about it. Yeah, the hurt is definitely there. I could really use some knee pads or a simple pillow. I could just grab a pillow from the living room couch. My couch is blue and I have many pillows on it. They showcase the colors I like. My favorite ones are branded with hues of red. They have been there for quite some time and have been very accepting of me and of my guests over the years. I mean, they literally opened up to all of those who squashed them with their backs, hugged them while sleeping, or simply used them for head and neck support. They are kind and work hard. I should probably let them be. But, what about my nagging knees? "Ah, just continue to dig", I tell myself. There is no need to participate in the drama. In fact, why even pause and stop the pain? Ditch the pillow! Forget it! Just dig. My nails are filled with dirt. I don't recognize my hands anymore. Maybe I should have worn gardening gloves. Probably not. Why create barriers against what feels so comforting? I want to touch anything that feels good and makes me want to scream, "This is it! This is what I want!" And, this is one of those moments when I get to scream really loud and perhaps louder: "I love!"

I am planting a rose bush. The buds will soon open. I need to dig this hole. Today! Now! I dig and dig. The soil feels cooler as I go deeper into the earth. Earthworms and grub worms scorn me for disrupting them. But that does not stop me. I am determined to go as deep as I can. I gently pick each worm with the tips of my fingers. I relocate them to a safe spot. I have nothing against them. It is the depths of the earth I am after. Have you ever looked closely down at the earth? I don't mean the hollow darkness that goes deeper and deeper. I mean, dig all you want. The scenery is pretty much the same. But, what if there was something worth looking at and feeling, reserved only for those who were willing to open up their minds and hearts? That is what I am after.

I am alone with my rose bush. I am holding it close to me. It's heavy but I will hold on to it as much as I can. It is like one of those countless times when I screamed, "I love!" I am now holding on to the rose bush because I can and I want to.

When I was a little girl, a boy ten years my senior taught me how to ride a bicycle in our neighborhood. That was the only real and meaningful interaction I had with him. Years later, when I became a college student, I accidentally met him at a wedding party. He remembered me but not the day he taught me how to ride a bicycle. I was heartbroken but still full of joy inside. I did not mean all that much to him but he meant the world to me. And, that was all I needed. I will always hold on to him like I am holding on to my rose bush.

I am back on my knees. The hole in the ground is big enough for my rose bush. It will grow tall and wide here. And, that's exactly what I want. I set it in the ground and slowly start backfilling. There is blood on my hands and arms but the dirt quickly covers the bleeding. This is what happens if you are not careful with the thorns.

Wasps are slowly building a nest in the gutter. They could not care any less about me or my rose bush. However, there will be others. I am reminded of how John Laroche, the American horticulturist in the movie adaptation of the book *The Orchid Thief*, passionately talks about bees and how they pollinate orchids: by simply doing what they are designed to do something large and magnificent happens. In this sense they show us how to live. How the only barometer you have is your heart. How when you spot your flower, you can't let anything get in your way. Healing is an everyday work-in-progress. My life's journey took its toll on me. I have seen the darkest side and the brightest side. Nothing is what it seems. Nothing. Sometimes the eyes speak, but you have got to have eyes of your own to see what is in the eyes of the other. Not everyone is qualified enough to do that. It takes courage and kindness. Some days I am in deep dark blue waters beyond anyone's imagination. I laugh it off. Other days, I fly high above the clouds. Nevertheless, I laugh it off as well. I always laugh it off. That's what I do. That's what I am good at.

My lawn is not green and manicured; it is a meadow. Earthworms and grub worms crawl underneath it. Moles chew on them. When it rains, birds probe for them with their thorny beaks. Every now and then, my blood fertilizes the soil. And I plant lots of rose bushes. As screenwriter Charlie Kaufman says: "You are what you love, not what loves you. That's what I decided a long time ago." I dig deep into the earth every chance I get. I am curious about what is beyond the deep hollow darkness. There is always something to see if you know how to look. And, my healing starts with each gaze as I look deeper into the hollow darkness, because that is where my rose bushes will survive and thrive. I don't let anything get in my way.

Daily Action Steps

- When you find yourself living in the past, wake yourself up to the right here, right now and simply place yourself in this very moment.
- When you find yourself living in the future, come back to the present by feeling the feelings now that you would like to feel later and then bask in the glory of the peace this brings to your now.
- Whatever you are doing right here, right now, whether it is filling you with fear, anxiety or anything troublesome, choose faith over worry in this very moment. Remember that you get to choose your thoughts.

About the Song "Back to The Garden"

When Maryann Ehmann invited me to sing and speak at her "Create Your Magnificent Year" event in 2015, she added me to the group e-mail she was sending out to the folks who were going to be attending her event. The wisdom Maryann shared in those emails got me so fired up that this song just came spilling out of me.

I am sharing this song with you here in hopes of inspiring you to live every moment, right here, right now.

Back to The Garden

Inspired by Maryann Ehmann & Marcus Slaton

Music & Lyrics by Janie Lidey, BMI

Time goes by and life rolls on
But every day is right here and is right now
Before it's gone

So I'm gonna live it out
I'm gonna sing and shout
And I'm gonna put my stake in the ground
I'm gonna dream as big as I can dream
Blazing from within
I'm gonna get myself back to the garden

I'm gonna fly so high and even if I fall
I'm not gonna fade away
I'm not gonna live my life as a flower on the wall

I'm gonna live it out
I'm gonna sing and shout
And I'm gonna put my stake in the ground
I'm gonna dream as big as I can dream
Blazing from within
I'm gonna get myself back to the garden

Round and round we go
Up and down and side to side
Spinning like a Ferris wheel
And sometimes it's like we're riding
On a wild and crazy rollercoaster ride

I'm gonna live it out
I'm gonna sing and shout
And I'm gonna put my stake in the ground
I'm gonna dream as big as I can dream
Blazing from within
I'm gonna get myself back to the garden...once again

CHAPTER #5

Believe in Your Angels

"If instead of a gem, or even a flower, we should cast the gift of a loving thought into the heart of a friend, that would be giving as the angels give."

~ George MacDonald ~

Do you ever feel like you are on your own? Do you ever wish that there were someone or something watching over you, maybe resting on your shoulder throughout your day? Angels are all around us and I believe that we all have a little bit of angel within us. We have the opportunity to be blessed by our angels and we also have the power to be an angel in someone else's life. Who is watching over you today and whose heart are you casting a loving thought into?

While traveling through California one summer, I ran into a lady in a laundry room after a day on the beach in sunny Santa Cruz. This lady turned her attention to me and asked me if I was having any female problems at the time. She said she noticed a certain dark aura coming from my lower abdomen. I thought it was an odd thing to be asked by a stranger, especially since I had actually been going through a series of medical procedures in that very area just before my trip. I said that I had and then I asked her what made her pose such a question. She said that she just had the gift of 'seeing' things. The next thing she said to me was that she sensed I was going through a rough period and that I must be some sort of writer who needed to experience the pain to gain the inspiration to write. Once again I thought it was an odd thing for a stranger to assume, especially since I had just finished writing an entire album worth of songs, all of which stemmed from the pain I was going through in this transition period of my life. I shared this with her and she just looked at me as if it all made perfect sense. It gets deeper...

My laundry room lady and I talked for a while and I shared with her that I had just spent the weekend in Newport Beach, California. I had gone down to attend a fund-raiser for a family friend named Amanda, who had been in a car accident and had slipped into a coma. A lot of the people at the benefit concert wore guardian angel pins in honor of Amanda in hopes that in doing so, we would be instrumental in helping her miraculously awaken from the state she was in. At this point in the story, the stranger stopped me and said that I had an angelic aura about me and that the next thing I wrote about should be angels. She said, "you need to know that this song isn't just for you and I mean that in a very big way!" "Truly," she stated, "big like Disney."

I flew back home to Alaska the next day and when I arrived, my piano lured me in. Out came a lovely song called, "Somethin' About An Angel"! I didn't feel like I really wrote the song myself. I was just the vessel as they say. One week later, I traveled south to Portland, Oregon for a voice care class and when asked to share something at the end of the week, I knew what song I had to sing. Moments after finishing my performance, two women came up to me, both in tears, and both with a story to tell. One woman said that she had decided not to attend this workshop after her son had died of AIDS that week but something kept drawing her toward the class. She said, "I think I am here because I was supposed to hear your song. It gave me so much hope and such a feeling of peace and I think it is the reason I came." The other lady, a new grandma, said that her daughter had just lost her child to SIDS and she was not doing well at all. She said that she felt like this song could save her daughter and could I please record it for her. I briefly thought back to the woman in the laundry room and wondered if this was what she meant when she said, "And you need to know that this song isn't just for you".

I flew back to Anchorage again with a new mission. I needed to find somewhere to record the angel song so that I could send it to these two women. While having a cup of coffee at a local coffee shop on my first morning back home, I imagined finding a recording studio that wasn't too expensive and maybe had a Christian type atmosphere. Moments later, a man I had met a few times before, came up and said hello to me. During our conversation, I brought up my desire to find a place to record and he just happened to have a friend that did some work out of his home. He mostly did Christian type projects and was priced reasonably.

It didn't take long to get hooked up with the recording engineer, as I was pretty much on fire by now. I set up a time to record and headed up to the studio. While recording the vocals for the angel song, I imagined that in the process of recording, the energy of it could be a cog in the wheel of Amanda, (the girl in the coma in Newport Beach) magically waking up. I brought the pencil drawing of Jesus that one of my high school students had given me that year, placed the picture on my music stand and while I sang, I prayed for Amanda to awaken from her coma. After I finished up with my recording project I decided to spend a night out with my girlfriends. At the end of the night, I played them my fresh new recording of the Angel song on the stereo in my Toyota 4-Runner. I told them the story about Amanda, the coma she was in, and the desire I had to help make a difference in her life through the energy of the angels and this song. The next morning, my friend Terri called me to ask if I had seen the story on CNN about the girl in Southern California who just miraculously came out of her coma over night! She of course said, "This can't be the girl you were telling us about! Can it?" I quickly phoned my sister Kris and was told that it *was* Amanda they were talking about on the news.

I believe that the hope, love and prayers that so many of us were sending out for Amanda created her miracle. We believed we would see and we did. Remember, the key to seeing miracles begins with believing that you will.

To believe in the things you can see and touch is no belief at all; but to believe in the unseen is a triumph and a blessing.

~ Abraham Lincoln ~

The Angel song came back into play again very soon after Amanda's miracle. I had been skiing at Mt. Alyeska just outside of Anchorage and ended up meeting a group of guys while taking a break and listening to the guitarist play in the lodge. One of the guys in the group had a little boy that was in Seattle at the Ronald MacDonald House, working on becoming a cancer survivor. The day after we all met, I decided to bring a copy of the Angel song over to the boy's father to share with his wife and family. I was hoping, of course, that it could have the same healing effect on their son, as it seemed to have had on Amanda. I am happy to share that the little boy is now a cancer free adult.

Over time, "Somethin' About an Angel" has continued to be a healing vessel for people all over the country. The kids in my choir heard the song and decided they wanted me to arrange a choral version of it for them to sing. Through the years, we were asked to sing it at funerals, World Aid's Day ceremonies, Veteran's Celebrations and more. I believe it helped the kids see the power we have to be of service to others through Love and kindness. We all have the power to be an angel for someone in need.

And now I'd like to introduce you to my dear friends, Dr. John Collins and his wife Tami. I have asked them to share their story with you here because when they heard of my diagnosis, they put on their angel wings and gifted me with ongoing complimentary weekly healing massage and advice on how the body heals.

Our Health Mission & Journey

Tami and I feel it is our job to educate and empower people to take control of their own health. And the good news is, your health is truly in your own hands.

In Alternative Healthcare we are taught that healing comes from within. Chiropractic philosophy teaches us that the innate intelligence of the body does not need any help, just no interference to do its job. The body is truly designed to heal, grow, and repair itself. Where there is life, there is the capacity for healing. For example, if you cut your finger and put a band-aid on it, a week later it is healed. What did the healing? Of course it was the body. If you cut the finger of a corpse and put a band-aid on it, a week later will it be healed? Of course not! So where does this healing ability arise from? It comes from within. It is the innate intelligence of the body. It is the life energy of the body. Some may refer to it as the body's spirit. This life energy knows exactly what is going on in the body at all times. It keeps you alive and does all the repair of the wear and tear of daily living.

Learning, reading, and studying about this wonderful healing ability of the body amazes and inspires me. It is what drives my passion to practice healthcare. But when I was a student in chiropractic school, I was perplexed at how wonderful the healing ability of the body is, yet how sick and in poor health the people of this world are. In 2017, we spent 18% of the Gross Domestic Product on healthcare. That was over ten thousand dollars per person in this country alone.

If our bodies are fearfully and wonderfully made as it is stated in Psalm 139:14, why are we experiencing such poor health? I could not fathom this incongruence. This burning question drove me to search for the answer. I found the answers from my teachers James Chestnut DC and Mark Hyman MD. Chiropractic Wellness and Functional Medicine teach that our health suffers and declines from the stressors that we experience in everyday life. These stressors are toxicities and deficiencies in how we eat, move, and think. To regain our health and vitality, we must provide purity and sufficiency in place of toxicity and deficiency to give the body the best ability to heal, grow, and repair itself.

Janie Lidey and her husband Sean have not only been patients at our office for over twenty years, they have been good friends. So when we received the news of Janie's diagnosis of stage IV breast cancer with metastasis to her bones, we were devastated. We asked, "How can this be...our Janie??" Janie was retired from the Anchorage School District and was living her heart's desire and dream. She was bringing her music to the world. She was so healthy, vibrant, and fit. Tami did her best to process this devastating news but it was very difficult for her. After crying many tears she decided she wanted to do something to help Janie. Tami wanted to give her the gift that could help with her healing. Instead of sending Janie flowers, she would give her a massage every week for as long as Janie felt that it was benefitting her. Tami's goal in using her massage, craniosacral therapy, and Reiki work, was to guide and support the innate intelligence to allow the healing to take place in Janie's body. Tami felt that she was the conduit from God/The Universe to guide the body back to the healing path.

Before each of her massage sessions with Tami, I counseled Janie on what to eat and just as important, when to eat. Fasting has been an ancient healing practice used around the world in every religion. Every week Janie and I would meet and discuss how she was doing with her diet and intermittent fasting. Every week seemed to bring good news on how she was feeling. She was feeling the love and care that Tami and I were pouring into her.

Just five short months after her diagnosis, Janie was declared cancer free. This time, the tears that Tami cried were tears of complete joy; the joy you feel when you are able to take your life's mission and use it to become an angel in someone's life. Like Janie said, "We all have the power to be an angel for someone in need."

Daily Action Steps

- Think of someone who might need an angel to come into their life and choose to cast the gift of a loving thought into their heart today.
- Put on your angel wings today and gift someone with your special angel energy.
- Open your heart to the angel resting on your shoulder today. (And if you think they will need to stay there for a while, wear something with padded shoulders.)

About the Song "Somethin' About an Angel"

This song came to life after having a discussion with a lady in a laundry room in California after a day on the beach in Santa Cruz. For some reason, she told me that I had an angelic aura about me and that the next thing I wrote about should be angels. She also said that the song wasn't just for me and that it was going to be big ~ like *Disney* big. A few days later, the song seemed to just write itself.

Many years have passed since this song was written and while in Nashville recording the songs for this project, a new version of it was born.

I am sharing this song with you here in hopes of inspiring you to believe that you are never alone, that your angels are surrounding you and that you have a powerful angel energy within you that can shine a guiding light on someone in need.

Somethin' About an Angel

Inspired by a myriad of Angels

Dedicated to the memory of Josh and Andrew Pepperd

Music & Lyrics by Janie Lidey, BMI &
Matt Wilder, ASCAP

There's somethin' about an angel
When your heart has fallen down
They'll lift you up they'll plant your feet
On solid ground
There's somethin' about an angel
When you've lost the strength to try
They'll make the wind lift up your wings
And give you flight

We don't always get to look our angels in the eye
And sometimes we're afraid
That they won't hear us when we cry
But if we open up our hearts
And let the Lord of angels in
He'll wrap us in their wings and help us fly again

Even without lookin' in their eyes
You will feel them standing by your side
They always lift you up so you can fly

They're your angels
They'll help you fly again

There's somethin' about an angel
When you're feelin' all alone
They'll take your hand they'll walk with you
They'll bring you home
So don't you ever forget your angels
When you thank your lucky stars
'Cause their magic lives within your heart
And they're always right there where you are

We don't always get to look our angels in the eye
And sometimes we're afraid
That they won't hear us when we cry
But if we open up our hearts
And let the Lord of angels in
He'll wrap us in their wings and help us fly again

Even without lookin' in their eyes
You will feel them standing by your side
They always lift you up so you can fly
They're your angels
They'll wrap you in their wings and help you fly again
They'll help you fly again

CHAPTER #6

Say Thank You

Gratitude is the healthiest of all human emotions. The more you express gratitude for what you have, the more likely you will have even more to express gratitude for.

~ Zig Ziglar ~

I am so grateful to be writing my gratitude chapter from the cushy seat of our new class A RV. My husband Sean, our son Tristan and our yellow lab Beaver are driving down the AlCan (Alaska/Canadian Highway) to launch Tristan into the next phase of his journey. He will be attending Embry-Riddle Aeronautical University in Prescott, Arizona and studying Astronautical Engineering. I am looking out a movie screen sized window: the perfect canvas on which to paint my thoughts about the magnificence of gratitude. As I share these thoughts, I am taking in the breathtakingly gorgeous views of Alaska and Canada. There are so many lakes and rivers that I have lost count. We have seen grizzlies, black bears, mama moose with twin babies, mountain goats and so many buffalo on some parts of the road that you could just barely squeeze through in the rig. Oh, and there go a small herd of caribou. I am filled with gratitude!

Being grateful is easy when everything is going your way. It is in times of adversity that you have to really dig deep to get to a place of thankfulness. When I choose to make gratitude one of my daily habits and I make it the first habit of my morning, it becomes easy to get to that thankful space regardless of what experiences come along on the journey. A diagnosis of stage IV metastatic breast cancer could have easily taken me to a very dark place. I could have wallowed in self-pity and gone through the *why me* syndrome. I could have cried my way through the phone calls I had to make to my family and friends. I could have gone immediately into fear and worry. Here is where the truth about gratitude comes in. While you don't always get to choose what happens to you, you certainly get to choose how you are going to react to what happens to you. I choose to react with gratitude. No matter how difficult the situation, goodness can always be found. What kind of goodness are you allowing to show up in your world today?

> *Gratitude is what we radiate when we experience grace, and the soul was made to run on grace the way a 747 runs on rocket fuel.*
>
> ~ John Ortberg ~

When my doctor Torrey Smith called me with the results of my MRI on that December morning in 2017, the first thing that came out of my mouth was a high pitched, "What?!" Cancer was the last thing in the world that I thought I would be diagnosed with. I had pain in my hip for several years and more recently in my lower back prior to the diagnosis and whenever I had those things checked out, the diagnosis was either sciatica or possibly some arthritis setting in. My family has a history of Osteoporosis so that too was a possibility. Cancer was never on the radar. But somehow, even in the midst of such a potentially devastating diagnosis, I was graced with a sense of gratitude.

Once again, I am convinced that the 8 daily habits I have chosen to live by are what allowed me to react to this potentially devastating news with grace and ease. After the shock of realizing this new normal in my life, I decided to begin feeling how grateful I would feel when I became cancer free and could call myself the miracle girl. I stepped into my new role as the Bionic Woman and began using my 8 daily habits to be the change I wanted to see in my healing journey. Here are the things that I focused on:

Habit #1: Act As If

I acted as if what I had been diagnosed with was just a bad bug that would melt away with the medications, radiation and surgery. And then I said Thank You.

Habit #2: Begin it Now

I began each day in gratitude, prayer and meditation. I started reading *A Daily Confession* by Charles Capps that a lovely lady named Jossie shared with me. I began watching some healing videos created by Ty Bollinger called, "The Truth About Cancer". I created a video series of my own called, "Cancer Unplugged", which sent a massive amount of Love out into the universe and in turn brought a whole lotta love back to me. I took up Qigong, which is a form of exercise that practices the art of energy work. I changed the things I put in my body and began the Ketogenic Diet. I created a shake that I am drinking daily that has organic frozen strawberries, blueberries, spinach and broccoli, fresh organic ginger and avocado, chaga mushroom, turkey tail mushroom extract, CBD powder, essential lemon oil, protein powder and some orange zero water. I began juicing with organic carrots, apples and ginger. I bought organic grass fed beef and made sure that everything I purchased to put in my body was free of hormones. I added lots of garlic to my diet. I began taking a drop of CBD oil each morning. I took up eating dark chocolate. I reduced my red wine intake to just one measured glass per evening. I started taking the following supplements recommended by my Naturopath: Vitamin K Full Spectrum, Coricepium, Multi-Nutrients 3, Pro Omega, Vitamin D3-5, Vitamin B shot, Magnesium Taurate, Ashwagandha, Taurine, Berberine, ResveraSirt-HP, Vitamin A, CuraMed and large doses of vitamin C. I also added Banyan Botanicals Healthy Hair to my daily supplements and although I have lost a lot of the hair on my body during this past year, I have been blessed with keeping the hair on my head. I began having a full body massage every week thanks to my dear friend Tami Collins. I listened to the special hypnotic healing recordings that my dear friend Suzy Prudden created just for me. And then I said Thank You.

Habit #3: Dream Big

I continued dreaming big about how this seemingly difficult time in my life would make me a stronger, more magnificent speaker, author and singer-songwriter and allow me the opportunity to be of service on a grander scale. And then I said Thank You.

Habit #4: Just Imagine

I imagined the old soul that I am and I called on her wisdom to heal my body. I also did some magnificent role-playing with my friend Glenn Morshower. Glenn is an actor, director and teacher, and one day while attending an event in LA, Glenn and I stood in the lobby and role-played the day that I got my new PET scan and found out I was cancer free. Just a few months later, it actually happened. And then I said Thank You.

Habit #5: Live in Gratitude

I spent loads of time just basking in gratitude. Gratitude for my deep conversations with Jesus. Gratitude for all of the healthy cells in my body. Gratitude for the time I was getting to spend with my family. Gratitude for how my husband Sean had become a magnificent caregiver. Gratitude for how canceling my concert load allowed me to spend more time at home with our son Tristan during his last semester of high school. Gratitude for the times I would just lay on our comfy bed with our yellow lab at my feet and do some inspirational reading. And then I said Thank You.

Habit #6: Let the Music Lift You

I let music raise my vibration by listening during meditations, driving, house cleaning and more. I played my guitar, piano, sang and wrote new songs. And then I said Thank You.

Habit #7: Laugh While You Leap

Sean became extra witty during this time and had me cracking up sometimes from the moment we woke up in the morning. I made sure to talk with my sisters, brother and mom a lot because for whatever reason, I seem to laugh harder with them than with anyone else. And then I said Thank You.

Habit #8: Leap with Love

I love Love. I have always loved Love. But during this time, I have grown an even keener sense for how Love heals. I am talking about Love on many levels. The Love of God, the Love of Jesus, The Love in our Universe, Loving our family, Loving our friends, Loving our Mother Earth, Loving ourselves, Loving the present moment, Loving our cells, Loving our journey, Loving what is... And then I said Thank You.

People who can be sincerely thankful for things which they own in imagination have real faith.

They will get rich; they will cause the creation of whatever they want.

~ Wallace Wattles ~

And now, I'd like to introduce you to my wonderful friend and Naturopath, Doctor Torrey Smith. I chose Torrey to be my special guest author in my gratitude chapter because he has so many great stories about helping people heal by teaching them the power behind sending thanks and love to parts of their body that need healing. I am so grateful for the team of doctors that Torrey gathered together to help usher me into wellness.

Thankful

Thankful. For all the hard working cells and life in our bodies. This was taught to me years ago by a patient who came to me plagued by a lifelong painful left leg. "I hate this leg," were her first words. Not only did it hurt all the time, but it also seemed to attract bad luck. "How?" I asked. It started with a bad rollover car wreck as a child, when her left leg was pinned. Then later her horse startled and fell over on her left leg. Several other accidents happened in her fifty years where her leg seemed to jump out and take the bullet. "Wow!" We both realized at once, the left leg had saved her life almost a dozen times. So, we decided to honor that hero leg and send all the loving energy possible every time it cried out with pain. Keeping it as clear as possible we settled on simply saying the word 'THANKFUL.' Warmth and regenerative blood flowed into it instantly and foe turned to friend. Her circulation opened up as the muscles relaxed from being tight and tense, which allowed a flood of loving energy to help her guardian angel leg to finally heal.

I try, often at a stop light while in a 'hurry' to get somewhere, to take time to thank my gut bacteria, my skin bacteria, and especially my mitochondria. The mitochondria are the power plants of our cells that come exclusively from the maternal line since the sperm mitochondria are destroyed in the fertilizing process. We are simply stewards for these life forms, and honoring them makes them glow. They are not used to being acknowledged and can get pretty excited to be recognized!

Each day is a gift, and I am grateful my patients continue to let me be a part of their journey to overcome obstacles so they can get on with their life destiny. Janie Lidey has been a great teacher for me on many levels and such a magnificent example of walking the talk. When the imaging came back of her leg showing it riddled with cancer, she embraced the shocking news and set about planning the next course of her life path. We put together a great team, all of whom were not only blown away by her optimism, but transformed by her desire to take this difficult news and plan how it could end up helping others. She was already out there spreading love through her songs and performances, but this took it to another level.

As we become closer to possible death we have one foot in heaven and one on the earth. Time goes into the 5th dimension when life becomes more precious. As a practitioner, and friend, we have the opportunity to have this bystander reaction just by being in the presence of this Godly connection. That may explain why some of the more gifted practitioners find working with those with life threatening disorders so fulfilling, since their patients are often more full of life and spirit than their complacent cousins.

Resonance: The ease of being at our most efficient. We have so much more to give away when we are in a resonant state. It is the classic example of gently running a moist finger over pure crystal glass producing a sonorous sound. Sitting and picturing every cell in our body vibrating at our own special frequency is a happy feeling. Not someone else's expectation, but simply just dialing in our own comfortable way of being. Resonant cells are healthy cells that use very little resources to do their work, which leaves an abundance of energy to give away. It is important to work on resonance first, then healing, then abundance, so that in giving, there is no debt created with the receiver.

Let your healthy cells teach the injured and cancerous cells to be good again. We thought we needed to kill the cancer cells but it may turn out they have lost their way, thrown off track by toxins and misguided influences and need to be reminded of the purity of their past. Good is greater than evil. Dr. Pollack, a biology professor at Columbia University, and Dr. Powers, now a cancer biologist at Cold Spring Harbor Laboratory and Stony Brook University, are spearheading the idea of 'reverting' cancerous cells back to normal cells! There are a number of herbs and nutrients that possibly work this way and at least one antidepressant medication that might be helpful. It is important to cross reference the effect of combining standard medical treatments with nutrients to assure there is synergism. Not surprisingly, there are many things that not only protect the good cells, but enable other treatments to work better at lower and less toxic doses.

Nurturing and nourishing the healthy cells and repairing the unhealthy cells is my primary goal as a naturopathic doctor. It takes a village to achieve wellness and balance, so while the oncologists are intent on knocking back the renegade cells, I focus on feeding the body, mind, and spirit to make the treatments work better with less damage. It is important to remember we are working with a person of destiny that has an illness, not an illness with a person attached. The ideal is that by giving the right attention to imbalances the patient will end up way healthier and happier than before hearing what began as devastating news.

People need to understand that as patients they hold the power in the room. Inspiration comes through them and then into the doctor (who if receptive, receives a bolt of celestial energy and knowledge particular to that special person). Getting the gift of the patient is something that feeds me daily. For inspiration I often put on one of Janie Lidey's CDs before starting my day and have to hold myself back from dancing on my desk from the excitement of partnering with that day's schedule of magnificent souls.

Daily Action Steps

- Before you even put your feet on the floor in the morning, spend time giving thanks for the blessings and miracles that you will experience in your day.

- Find a way to say more thank yous than usual to people you encounter while journeying through your day. It will lift them up but it will also help you fly a little higher.

- When you lay down to go to sleep at night, give thanks for the blessings that showed up in your day and also for how you were able to be a light in someone else's darkness.

About the Song "Thank You"

The inspiration behind this song came from my amazing friend Stephanie Adriana Westover. She mentioned one day that it would be so perfect if I were to write a "Thank You" song, because gratitude is so big in the world right now and it is so much a part of how we each live our lives. The night before she told me that, I literally was dreaming about a "Thank You" song I sang back in college and then later taught to my choirs. It seemed like a sign, and soon after, this song came along.

I am sharing this song with you here in hopes of inspiring you to believe that when you choose to live in gratitude throughout your day, your life will be filled with more things to be grateful for.

Thank You

Inspired by Stephanie Adriana Westover

Music & Lyrics by Janie Lidey, BMI

T H A N K Y O U — T H A N K Y O U

If you say these two words
Before you even put your feet on the floor
You will wake up on the right side of your bed
Like never before
And if you say these two words
Before you close your eyes and turn out the light
You will wake up in the morning
Feeling like you grew a set of wings overnight

Thank you for a good night's sleep
Thank you for the air I breathe
Thank you for the morning sun
Thank you for a day of fun

My feet don't even touch the ground for the day
Until I take the time to say

T H A N K Y O U — T H A N K Y O U

When I lay me down to sleep for the night
I say a prayer
In thanks for everything that's going so right
And then I dream of all the possibilities
That I know tomorrow tomorrow holds for me

Thank you for a good night's sleep
Thank you for the air I breathe
Thank you for the morning sun
Thank you for a day of fun

My feet don't even touch the ground for the day
Until I take the time to say

T H A N K Y O U – T H A N K Y O U

Thank you for a good night's sleep
Thank you for the air I breathe
Thank you for the morning sun
Thank you for a day of fun

CHAPTER #7

Thrive and Survive

For every wound there is a scar, and every scar tells a story. A story that says, "I Survived!"

~ Craig Scott ~

It used to be that when I would think about what a survivor was, I would think about someone who had been through a battle with cancer, survived chemo and radiation and was now hoping to live a long and healthy life. And the thing is, so many of us know someone who has done just that. But over time, I have realized that we are all survivors of one thing or another. Be it cancer or any other challenge in life, we all have a reason to say, "I'm a Survivor!" What are you surviving in your life today?

When people meet me, they usually think I am someone who is happy, healthy and living a blessed life. Happy, yes! Blessed, yes! Healthy? I am now, but when it comes down to it, I have been diagnosed with Epstein Bar, had my tonsils removed, my uterus yanked, my bladder tucked, my herniated umbilical fixed, cranial surgery for a depressed skull fracture after putting a ski through my head, twelve inches of my intestine removed due to chronic Diverticulitis and a stage IV metastatic breast cancer diagnosis that left me with a titanium rod in my right femur among other things. I have a hard time imagining that I have survived all of those things but now more than ever I have reason to say, "I'm a Survivor!"

Several years ago I was asked to sing for a Cancer Relay in California's Bay Area. The committee had requested that I sing a cancer survivor song that Melissa Etheridge had sung after her cancer diagnosis. But when I tried to learn it, it just wasn't something that fit my voice. At that time, my dad was surviving prostate cancer, my brother-in-law was surviving testicular cancer, and my cousin was working on becoming a breast cancer survivor. As I thought about what they were all going through and what we as family members who deeply loved them were going through, I realized we were all becoming survivors on some level and that we were surviving because of the love we were infusing into one another. All of these feelings inspired me to write a new survivor song and the committee for the Cancer Relay decided that my song fit the event better than the one they had originally requested. After singing the song for the Relay in California, I was asked if it could be used for a PSA to advertise the Alaska Run for Women. This was followed by an opportunity to sing the song in front of two thousand women at the start of the race in Anchorage that year. As I stood and sang to this group of beautiful women, the Love radiating from their hearts and mine could have lit up the whole planet. Some of these women had cancer, and some were running in support of those with cancer. Some of these women wore wigs because they had lost their hair, and some were wearing wigs in support of those who had lost their hair. Unconditional love was flowing through this group and its energy was helping us all not only survive, but thrive.

> *When the Japanese mend broken objects, they aggrandize the damage by filling the cracks with gold. They believe that when something's suffered damage and has a history it becomes more beautiful.*
>
> ~ Barbara Bloom ~

Several years later, while in Nashville recording some new material, I was asked to do a re-make of the survivor song. The timing seemed amazingly right, considering my niece had recently become a survivor, my cousin had just been diagnosed with Lymphoma, one of my dear Nashville friends was going through chemotherapy and my producer, who is now my co-writer on this project, was a cancer survivor himself. When I first wrote the song, I was not a cancer survivor. When I did the re-mix of the song, I was not a cancer survivor. I have decided to do a new re-mix of the song because this time, when I sing the lyrics, I will be singing them as a true cancer Survivor. I am a survivor because I choose to *Expect Blessings and Miracles.* I am a survivor because I choose to *Radiate Hope.* I am a survivor because I choose to *Fly High.* I am a survivor because I choose to *Be Present.* I am a survivor because I choose to *Live in Gratitude.* I am a survivor because I choose to *Believe in My Angels.* I am a survivor because I choose to *Thrive & Survive.* And I am a survivor because I choose to *Radiate Love.*

And now, I'd like to introduce you to my dear friend and Nashville producer, Matt Wilder. He too is a cancer survivor and co-writer on many of my album projects. Working with Matt has brought me to a whole new level as a songwriter and musician.

Second Chances

As Janie's Nashville producer, I've had the pleasure of watching her create and discover her own sound. All along, her genuine positivity has been her trademark. It's funny, but when Janie first shared her cancer diagnosis with me, I never thought of her as "unhealthy". On some level, I believe everything that ever was, or ever will be, is contained in the eternal "present". I just felt she was going to be okay.

I too am a cancer survivor. I try not to think about what I went through eleven years ago, except as a reminder to be thankful every day of my life going forward. Ultimately, my story is a tale of redemption and second chances. The loss of virtually everything followed by a rebirth and a better life. You really never know what's going to happen on this journey and it is in times of adversity that we awaken to a deeper purpose.

After nearly twenty years of marriage and raising two beautiful children, I began to wake up to the emotional desert my life had become. I never felt truly loved and it seemed as though my love was never really wanted or accepted. Something was missing and that stress had taken a considerable toll on me through the years. At the age of forty-five, my wife and I decided to go our separate ways. Before moving forward, I decided to see if I had a clean bill of health and scheduled a colonoscopy. When I was twenty-six my mother died from colon cancer after a valiant fight, and my older brother had polyps removed in recent years so I just wanted to check things out before moving on.

On the day of my colonoscopy, I was actually awake during the first part of the procedure and remember seeing the growth in my colon before I passed out. The reality and significance of this did not sink in until the doctor came into recovery and said, "I'm afraid you have cancer."

Sometimes when it rains it pours and over the course of the next few months I would see the end of my marriage, start the fight for my life and endure the loss of my job on top of it all. The possibility of death is scary, but my biggest fear was that I might never know the kind of love or marriage my parents had before I died. They had set an example of what a marriage could be and I did not want this to be the end of the road for me. I am so grateful for the presence of my mother's spirit at that time in my life, as it gave me great faith and hope while becoming the survivor that I am today.

I was a Rockstar at getting back on my feet after my surgery and before I knew it, I was home from the hospital recovering. However, after a couple of days, my health began to deteriorate and I became so sick that I could no longer get out of bed. Fortunately, at my daughter's request, our neighbor and nurse Laura Winslow came by and immediately took me to the emergency room. She saved my life that day. While in the hospital, my biopsy results came back and I learned that very little of my growth was cancerous and since it was stage I, it would not even require chemo. That was the good news. The bad news was that I would have to go back into surgery because my intestines had tangled and were no longer connected together when the doctor opened me up. If I hadn't been taken to the hospital that day, I may not have survived. Following the surgery, I experienced several days of the most intense pain imaginable. The strongest dosage of Morphine could hardly put a dent in it. It was like having hundreds of knives plunged into my belly over and over again without a break and I watched every tick of every second on the clock telling myself "this will pass. It will get better if I can just hang on". I prayed to God to let me live so that I could one day experience the love I longed for.

My prayers were answered when nine months into my recovery I was introduced to my future wife. Suddenly I was thrust into a new life. Sometimes it is in our darkest moments that we are brought into the light.

At the time of this writing I've lived eleven years cancer free. I have had ten glorious years in a loving marriage with my beautiful wife Kerstin and we have been blessed with two amazing children. I am living the life I dreamed of and whenever my time comes I will leave this earth a far happier man for what I have been through. I am a survivor and for that I am grateful with all my heart every day of my life. My prayers were answered. Sometimes we get second chances.

Daily Action Steps

- Take some time each day to send Love to your cells and thank them for all they are doing to help you thrive and survive.

- When you find out that you have something going on in your body that is out of sync with your wellness, choose to radiate hope and love into yourself.

- If you have an illness, remember that you have the power of healing within you. You get to choose to thrive and survive and your positivity about your situation can bring about Blessings and Miracles.

About the Song "Survivor"

Survivor started out as a song called, *Because of the Love.* It is the song I talked about earlier that I wrote for the Cancer Relay in California. Since then it has had a few remakes and this version of it is what was born after I became a cancer survivor.

I am sharing this song with you here in hopes of inspiring you to believe that you are not alone and that being a survivor has so much to do with choosing to be thankful for each breath along the way and for all the Love that is in your life, every single day.

Survivor

Inspired by Faith, Hope & Love
Music & Lyrics by Janie Lidey, BMI &
Matt Wilder, ASCAP
©2018

Another day has come and gone
A brand new miracle the chance to sing my song
From my knees Lord I have prayed for another day
Life can take you by surprise

Another day I'm standing here
I've crossed so many miles and faced so many fears
And I've been more than shaken
On this road I've taken
But Lord I've come to realize

I'm a survivor and I'm not alone
I'm a survivor I never give up hope
I'm a survivor truly inspired one thing
I know that I'm older and wiser
Is somehow I am gonna make it home
I'm a survivor I'm a survivor

No more moments filled with doubt
'Cause now I know just how the story will turn out
When the slope was steep and rocky

Climbing with a broken body
I took it one step at a time

I'm a survivor and I'm not alone
I'm a survivor I never give up hope
I'm a survivor truly inspired one thing
I know that I'm older and wiser
Is somehow I am gonna make it home
I'm a survivor

Thankful for each breath I take
Each friend along the way
For all the love that's in my life
For every single day

I'm a survivor never give up hope
I'm a survivor truly inspired one thing
I know that I'm older and wiser
Is somehow I am gonna make it home
I'm a survivor I'm a survivor I'm a survivor
I'm a survivor

CHAPTER #8

Radiate Love

Even after all this time the sun never says to the earth, "You owe me." Look what happens with a love like that. It lights the whole sky.

~ Hafiz ~

During the past year, more than ever, I have come to realize the importance of choosing Love over fear. We are all extraordinary beings and it is our choice to be so from the moment we realize our first breath of the day. We have the power to light up the world by Radiating Love. Just imagine what can happen with a Love like that.

You know that feeling you get when your eyeballs first pop open for the day and you become aware of something that happened the day before that was really difficult? Maybe there was a cancer diagnosis, a death in the family, a bad car wreck or any number of things that life can offer up. There is that moment of peace, maybe only seconds, where you haven't recalled the memory of the prior day yet, and then WHAM! It hits you like an elephant sitting on top of your chest and squeezing the blood out of your body, making it very hard for you to gulp in enough air to keep you alive. During that moment of becoming aware, you have a choice. You can choose fear or you can go directly to Love. You get to choose your thoughts. What are you choosing to think about first thing in your morning?

I have heard fear described as False Evidence Appearing Real and Love described as Living One Vibrational Energy. When we commit to Radiating Love and Living One Vibrational Energy, we give ourselves the power to close the door on fear. We are all instruments of peace. Within us lies the power to be Love, the power to heal, the power to shine a brighter light than we knew we were capable of shining. As I shared with you in the beginning of our journey through *Radiating Hope ~ Cancer Unplugged,* the key to seeing miracles begins with believing that you will. The key to being blessed begins with believing that you are. Let's add to that, the key to Radiating Love begins with believing in the brightness of your light.

> *The more we truly desire to benefit others, the greater the peace and happiness we experience. Through Love, through kindness, through compassion we establish understanding between ourselves, and others. This is how we forge unity and harmony.*
>
> ~ Dalai Lama ~

In this final chapter of *Radiating Hope ~ Cancer Unplugged,* I would like to challenge you to wake up each day and go directly to Love. Love of Source, Love of God, Love of Jesus, Love of Angels, Love of Universal Energy, Love of Self, Love of Family, Love of your Dog or anything else that makes you feel that sense of peace and calm to your very core. How you start your day has everything to do with how your day goes.

One of the things that I have come to realize more than ever during this time of change in my life is that when I do something loving for someone else, it is that which creates my own happiness and consequent healing. When I started creating my *Cancer Unplugged* videos, I did so because a lot of people were feeling sadness when they heard the news of my diagnosis and I wanted them to know that I was okay. I wanted to find a way to create a feeling of hope for my family, friends, fans and former students. I started including one of my original songs in each video because, remember, my big childhood dream was to raise the vibration of love on our planet with my music. I wanted to lift people up and send out a loving message that I knew would create a feeling of peace about what was happening to me. I began to realize more than ever that my peace and happiness was heightened by the peace and happiness I was able to create for others.

One day, upon finishing one of the songs for my new book, I had this incredibly strong feeling that I should find a way to share the song *Radiating Hope* with my radiation oncologist Dr. Larry Daugherty. Larry, along with my brother in law Dave McHone, had inspired me to write the song. I kept hearing this whisper that I should go into Larry's office and play the song for him. And then I would allow fear to creep in and dismiss that whisper, thinking that it was silly for me to interrupt him during his busy workday. I spent the better part of the next morning hearing the God whisper and then talking myself out of doing it. I remember going back and forth with the voice in my head. The voice of Love would say that I should do this because it will lift and inspire Larry to hear the song. The voice of fear would say I should just wait and let him hear it when the book and companion CD was a finished product. I knew that I would be recording the song in Nashville and I began to think that maybe it would be better for him to hear the final version than for me to share it with him in raw form. And besides, Larry was such a happy guy, why would I need to lift and inspire him?

What happened next was such a lovely reminder of the importance of listening to the whisper. I suddenly had this overwhelming feeling that there was a reason I was hearing God's voice and I packed up my guitar and headed for the clinic. I had emailed Larry when the whisper began the day before to let him know that I might be dropping by and he said he could break away for a few minutes. I arrived at the Alaska Cancer Treatment Center that morning with a yearning in my heart to simply make a positive difference in someone's world with one small act of kindness.

Larry and I sat at the conference table in his office and I shared with him that the song had been inspired by him, his *Radiating Hope* Foundation and the climb that my brother in law Dave McHone had made to deliver my prayer flag to the top of Mt. Kilimanjaro. While singing the song, Larry got rather emotional and when I finished, he said that this was one of the kindest acts that he had witnessed in his life. He said it couldn't have happened at a more profound moment in his life. What he told me next was nothing short of a miracle. That very morning, Larry's mentor, Luther Brady, had passed away. Luther had been influential in helping Larry create his *Radiating Hope* Foundation among many other things. And here I was singing him this song on the very day that Luther got his promotion to Heaven. I shared with him that I almost talked myself out of visiting him that day because, after all, why would someone like Larry need lifting up. I am so glad that I chose Love over fear that morning. Had I gone with fear, I wouldn't have known about Luther, his influence on the *Radiating Hope* Foundation and his passing that day. Because I chose Love, the song is now dedicated to Luther's memory. I have heard it said that God's one and only voice is silence. It's the silence between the notes that makes the music.

> *There are only two days in the year that nothing can be done. One is called yesterday and the other is called tomorrow. Today is the right day to love, believe, do and mostly live.*
>
> ~ Dalai Lama ~

And now I'd like to introduce you to my buddy and founder of *Dave, the Caregiver's Caregiver,* Dave Nassaney. I asked Dave to be my special guest author for this chapter because his is a story of how love can radiate with a power capable of lifting you out of your darkest moment and into your brightest light. I have had the pleasure of becoming dear friends with Dave and his lovely bride Charlene and have been awakened by the light illuminating from Charlene's eyes.

A Love Story

My wife Charlene and I had a fairy-tale courtship, romance, and marriage for the first twenty-one years of our lives together. We were so much in love that I just had to marry this beautiful, blue-eyed wonder, who would look down into my soul every time she pierced into my eyes and saw the good in me that I didn't even realize existed myself.

I never wanted to marry anyone, because I was a confirmed bachelor. But after only fifteen months of dating Charlene, I could not imagine life without her. I was having second thoughts about my philosophy on marriage. We never argued, or disagreed on anything. I also didn't want to kick myself in the butt for the rest of my life for letting such a gem get away from me.

We broke up to consider what life would be like without each other. Three days later, we both had to reunite because we could not fathom life without the other. We married in ten short days.

After raising our three daughters, getting them all married off and out of the house, we became excited and happy empty-nesters. Life was good. We traveled a lot and enjoyed our freedom. Then one morning, Charlene complained of a bad headache that she'd been having for three days. We didn't pay much attention to it at first, but then, on the fourth morning, the headache ceased being *only* a headache. By the time the ambulance arrived, it was too late. The woman I loved had suffered a massive stroke that left her severely speech impaired and paralyzed on the right side. Our world immediately turned upside down. Our lives have never been the same.

Instead of entering the empty-nest phase of life that we had always looked forward to, I found myself having to constantly care for the love of my life 24/7. There is no way that anyone can ever prepare for that. To be honest, the first two years were a living hell for us. I didn't know what I was doing. I didn't know how to care for my wife. Charlene became angry and bitter because she was no longer the woman that she was before. I became angry and bitter for the same reasons. I grieved that my wife was no longer the woman that I married. I still loved her, but it was very hard being on the receiving end of her anger brought about by her grief. I felt so guilty. In fact, I came to a point that I didn't know if I could do it any longer. One day, I sat down and wrote her a letter: "Charlene, you are so mean to me. It's so hard being your husband taking care of you all the time without feeling *any* love in return. I just don't know if I can be with you any longer. I'll take care of you financially, but I can't be with you." I read that letter over and over again, but I just couldn't give it to her. I *wanted* to love my wife. I *wanted* to care for her, but it seemed impossible. I really didn't know *how* to care for my wife anymore. I didn't know if I even *wanted* to. I wondered if there was any hope for us.

Then one day, I found a card in my pocket inviting me to a caregiver's support group. I didn't even know what a caregiver was but I figured if someone gave it to me, maybe I should go. Going to that group changed everything for me. I found hope again and I discovered that I had to take care of me before I could take care of my wife. They tell us on airplanes that in the event of an emergency, we are to put *our* oxygen mask on first *before* we attempt to help our loved ones with their masks. That's such a great metaphor for all of life: Take care of you *first*, not out of selfishness, but out of survival.

When I finally realized how much I was able to change, to my surprise, my wife also changed. I was no longer thinking about how she made me feel. I was just taking care of me, so I could take care of her. After two years, Charlene finally reached the acceptance stage of her grief, and she became her old self again. I am very proud of her. She was, and still is, a cross between Martha Stewart and Wonder Woman. She makes us "normal" people look like whiners and complainers. She is my hero!

Because of my experience, I realized that there are so many other caregivers out there all going through this incredible pain, feeling lost and alone, and I wanted to help them triumph over that pain. I didn't want them to give up like I almost gave up. That's why I became *Dave, the Caregiver's Caregiver.*

Janie asked me to share my story in the final chapter of her book because of the blessings and miracles that have transpired in my life through love and hope. She has seen the power of love and hope radiate from the eyes of my beautiful Charlene and witnessed the pure goodness that can come to us when we care deeply enough to take care of ourselves first and in doing so, become a light in someone else's darkness.

Daily Action Steps

- When your eyeballs pop open for the day, take time to Radiate Love. Breathe in the Love of God, the Love of Jesus, the Love of Angels, the Love of the Universe or anything else that inspires you. As you breathe out, send your Love into the world. You can be as specific as you want with this. If there isn't someone or something you want to focus on then simply allow your Love to permeate whatever space it naturally flows out to.

- Have a stack of note cards on hand and when you get up out of bed, grab your pen and jot a note of Love to someone who may need a little Love infusion.

- When you make breakfast or lunches for yourself or your family, infuse them with Love as you make them. I believe that when we radiate Love into our food during preparation, it will not only taste better, it will be healthier to eat.

- If you have pets in your household, Love on them a little extra as you head out for the day.

About the Song "Take a Leap of Love"

After attending a leadership event with Larry Broughton and Craig Duswalt in Los Angeles in 2016, I couldn't wait to get back to my hotel room on the final night. I wanted to gather my notes from our two days together and put together a song that captured the essence of our time together. "Take a Leap of Love" is what came to me that night.

I am sharing this song with you here in hopes of inspiring you to believe that it is who you are, not what you are that matters. You can be the miracle in someone else's day when you choose to Radiate Love.

Take a Leap of Love

Inspired by Larry Broughton & Craig Duswalt
Music & Lyrics by Janie Lidey, BMI &
Matt Wilder, ASCAP

It's who you are not what you are lean into your gift
Always lead with kindness
This is the life you came here to live
Decide to be the miracle in someone else's day
It's time to make the magic happen
In the Disney kind of way

Let your voice be heard let your hands reach out
Fill someone with hope 'cause hope is what it's all about
Shine your brightest light and you will rise above
Give all you can give take the leap of Love

It's who you are not what you are
That's where it all begins
You put your wheels in motion
And the journey never ends
Decide to be the miracle in someone else's day
It's time to make the magic happen
In the Disney kind of way

Let your voice be heard let your hands reach out
Fill someone with hope 'cause hope is what it's all about
Shine your brightest light and you will rise above
Give all you can give take the leap of Love

Take the leap of Love take the leap of Love
Take the leap of Love take a leap

Let your voice be heard let your hands reach out
Fill someone with hope 'cause hope is what it's all about
Shine your brightest light and you will rise above
Take the leap of Love take the leap of Love
Take the leap the leap of Love

Afterword

I believe that when you choose to *Expect Blessings and Miracles,* you will see them come to life daily. Remember that the key to being blessed begins with believing that you are. The key to seeing miracles begins with believing that you will. I believe that when you choose to *Radiate Hope,* you will not only create wellness for yourself, you will infuse others with it as well. I believe that when you choose to *Fly High,* you will find that the universe supports your dreams with unlimited power and alignment. I believe that when you choose to *Be Present,* you are more likely to experience Love over fear and faith over worry. I believe that when you choose to *Remember your Angels,* you will float through your days with ease knowing that whatever comes along, you are not alone. I believe that when you choose to *Say Thank You,* you will see more things come into your life to make you grateful. I believe that when you choose to *Thrive and Survive,* you will ignite the quiet power of the universe to cheer you on. And I believe that when you choose to *Radiate Love,* the vibration of your love will light up the universe.

May you expect Blessings and Miracles, may you choose Love over fear and faith over worry, may you use your gifts to benefit others and may you Radiate Hope!

Love Janie

2018

About the Song "Foreverville"

The Love I feel for my husband Sean and our son Tristan has brought me to a place of knowing that a Love like that doesn't just go away when we leave this place. It is an ingredient that will continue to be used in the mix for all of eternity. When I think of eternity, I think of a state of mind where I exist in a pool of Love. I like to call that place Foreverville.

I am sharing this song with you here in hopes of inspiring you to believe in the hope of an infinite tomorrow, a state of mind where Love lives on in Foreverville.

Foreverville

Inspired by Sean & Tristan Lidey

Music & Lyrics by Janie Lidey, BMI, Tristan Lidey & Matt Wilder, ASCAP

It was the spring of '98 was it luck or was it fate
You weren't even supposed to be there on that day
I fell deep and you fell hard
Like we were written in the stars
I was about to leave but then I stayed

In a world of ifs and maybes
You locked me in for good with just one look
Fleeting moments and temporaries
Just a wink in time was all it took
To know I'd love you to Foreverville...

Time goes by and life goes fast
Ya wonder if love's gonna last
'Cause it can be a hard climb up the hill
We grow old and then we die
And somebody's gotta stay behind
And a broken heart can make it hard to keep on tryin'
Unless you know somebody... is waiting for you

In Foreverville...
In Foreverville...
Forever

The sun was golden in the sky
It's how we caught each other's eye
And before we knew the moon was flyin' high
It was our very first hello and we never said goodbye
'Cause Foreverville is beyond the end of time

In a world of ifs and maybes
You locked me in for good with just one look
Fleeting moments and temporaries
Just a wink in time was all it took
To know I'd love you to Foreverville...

Time goes by and life goes fast
Ya wonder if love's gonna last
And it can be a hard climb up the hill
We grow old and then we die
And somebody's gotta stay behind
And a broken heart can make it hard to keep on tryin'
Unless you know somebody... is waiting for you
In Foreverville...
In Foreverville...
Forever

Encore: Bonus Track just for the fun of it.

About the Song "A New Rod and Reel"

For many years I have shared a story and song with my audiences about a gift I wished for on our ten-year anniversary. Sean and I had been fishing one day in Alaska and it suddenly dawned on me that he had an awfully spiffy titanium rod and two-speed reel and I was sitting there with an old, heavy 1960's halibut rod. We were coming up on our ten-year anniversary and Sean asked me, "Hey sweetie, what do you think you want for our ten-year?" He was thinking I might want diamonds or pearls but I said, "Heck no, I want a new rod and reel!"

I am sharing this with you here at the end of our time together in hopes of inspiring you to always keep a good sense of humor about what happens to you in your life. I just find it rather funny that I have been telling the story of wishing for a new titanium rod for years, and while I did get that fishing pole back in the day, I now have a new titanium rod in my right femur. I guess ya have to be careful what you wish for!

A New Rod and Reel

Inspired by Sean Lidey

Music & Lyrics by Janie Lidey, BMI

©2010

We'd been together for almost ten years
Filled with laughter and lovin' and just a few tears
When my baby asked me what I wanted for our ten
And my answer made him fall for me all over again

Ya see most girls want diamonds or fresh water pearls
But I just ain't one of them girly girls
What I want is made of titanium and steel
Baby I want a new rod & reel

When we got to fifteen he asked me again
What'd make me happy like I was at our ten
And I said my waders were leaking and so
Could he buy me some new ones and off we would go

Ya see most girls want diamonds or fresh water pearls
But I just ain't one of them girly girls
What I want is made of titanium and steel
Baby I want a new rod & reel

When we hit our twenty he looked me in the eye
He said I guess that it's time again to go out and buy

He asked me what I really wanted a lot
I said Baby I think I've earned a yacht

So that we can go fishin' and use them old boots
And the rod that ya gave me when mine went kaput
And right then he led me outside our back door
And there was my new fishin' boat just sittin' on shore

Ya see most girls want diamonds or fresh water pearls
But I just ain't one of them girly girls
What I want is made of titanium and steel
Baby I want a new rod & reel
Baby I want a new rod & reel

CD Info for the Music in *Radiating Hope*

Go to janielidey.com for information
on ordering your CD.

Each chapter in *Radiating Hope* ends with an original song that connects to the message in the story. Music has a way of raising our vibration and lifting us higher. It is my prayer that these songs will give you an additional boost in radiating hope into your life. You can listen to samples of the songs on my website and then either order your CD directly from janielidey.com or find me on iTunes, Amazon, CD Baby, and more ...

I would like to thank the musicians who contributed to the production of this CD. They have all helped me rise to a higher standard on my journey as a musician, and beyond their remarkable musical talents, they are some of the kindest, most compassionate human beings on the planet. Their presence on this project is one of my big Blessings and Miracles.

Matt Wilder—Producer, Backup Vocals, Keyboard & Guitar

Joey Turner and Casey Wood—Additional Engineering

Mike Brignardello, Joeie Canaday & Gary Lunn—Bass

Jenee Fleenor—Fiddle, Guitar, Mandolin & Backup Vocals

Jimmy Nichols—Keyboards
Jerry Kimbrough—Acoustic & Electric Guitar
Janie Lidey—Lead Vocals, Backup Vocals & Acoustic Guitar
Lonnie Wilson—Drums

~ To View Janie's *Cancer Unplugged* Videos ~
Visit her youtube channel.

https://www.youtube.com/c/JanieLideyMusic

Janie created her Cancer Unplugged Videos to share:

- A message of Hope and Healing
- Original Music that will Lift and Inspire
- Thoughts about how she went from a stage IV metastatic breast cancer diagnosis to being cancer free in just 5 short months

About the Author

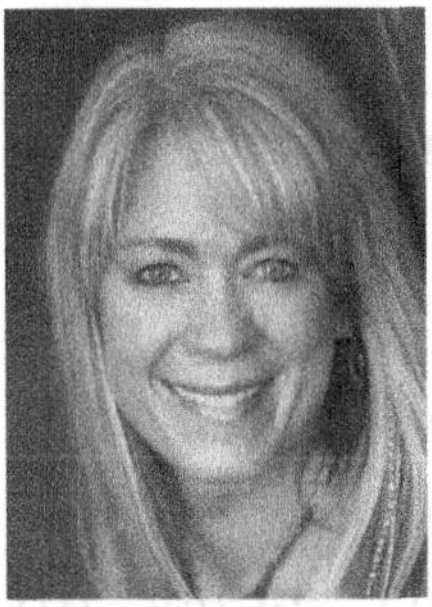

Janie Lidey is a dynamic speaker, best selling author, Emmy winning songwriter and Grammy winning music educator who dedicated herself to teaching music in the public schools of Alaska for twenty-six years. She started out teaching music in remote, fly-in-only villages, and in 2011, after seventeen years as the choir director and guitar teacher at Grammy Award winning East High School, Janie stepped out of the safety and comfort of one school to make the world her classroom.

Lidey has been recognized for her excellence through winning an Emmy for her songwriting; a Grammy for the fine arts program she helped direct at East High School in Anchorage, Alaska; the Mayor's Arts Award, which recognizes excellence in music education; and a spot on the George Lucas Edutopia website for her role in helping make the world a better place. Mrs. Lidey not only taught her students to sing and play the guitar, she taught them to live their lives with passion, kindness, love, hope, and gratitude. The most important lesson was to instill the belief in her students that they could be or do anything they dreamed or imagined. Seeing the effect she was having on her students throughout the years made Janie feel a responsibility to step out and contribute on a global level.

Janie speaks and sings to audiences across the country, inspiring them to create the life they have only dared to dream about. Some of her favorite events have been Craig Duswalt's *Rock Your Life Night* in Anaheim, California, Natasha Duswalt's *Women Who Rock Event* in Los Angeles, California; *Author 101 University* in Southern California; *Rachel's Challenge Summit* (Columbine tragedy) in Denver, Colorado; Women's Conferences in Alaska, California, and Iowa and Cancer Relays along the West Coast and Alaska. She also had the opportunity to perform along with John Carter Cash at Willie Nelson's eightieth birthday tribute in Nashville, Tennessee.

Janie has lived in Alaska for over thirty years. She taught music in eight remote, fly-in-only villages; was a fork- lift operator for a salmon fishery in Bristol Bay (where she occasionally sang and played her guitar in the saloon during fish closures); skied double black diamond, expert-only ski runs; paraglided off Hatcher Pass; ran a Segway tour business around Lake Hood and built her own log home with her husband, Sean, where they have lived together with their son, Tristan, for seventeen years. They share their yard with an occasional mama and baby moose, black bear, brown bear, and lynx, but their favorite four-legged friend is their big yellow lab, Beaver.

In 2017, Janie was diagnosed with stage IV metastatic breast cancer. When the doctors told her that it was incurable, Janie told them that didn't work for her. Just five months after the diagnosis, Janie was cancer free!

She is using her miracle story and her music to infuse hope, love, and light into her audiences.

www.janielidey.com

About Janie's Special Guest Authors

Gene Ehmann

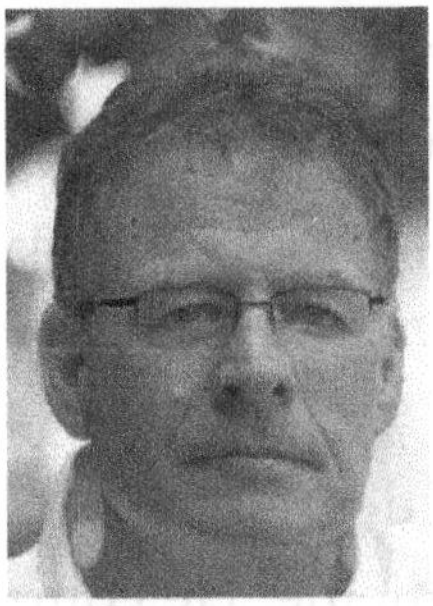

Gene Ehmann was born in Long Beach, California and graduated from Cal State University, Long Beach. He earned his Master's from University of Arizona and his Doctorate in Ministry from Bethany Divinity College and Seminary.

Gene has served a myriad of posts including Long Beach Police Officer; Special Agent, FBI; and Director of Rocky Mountain Information Network, State of Arizona. He led the investigation on Joseph Bonanno, head of Mafia, the prototype of the God Father as portrayed in the movie.

Gene has been a Private Investigator since 1980 and is currently an Investigator of counterfeit products. He has traveled in over 25 countries investigating and providing Executive Security. Locally, he investigates a wide variety of matters.

Gene is married and is the father of 4 children, 11 grandchildren, and 2 great grandchildren.

Larry Daugherty

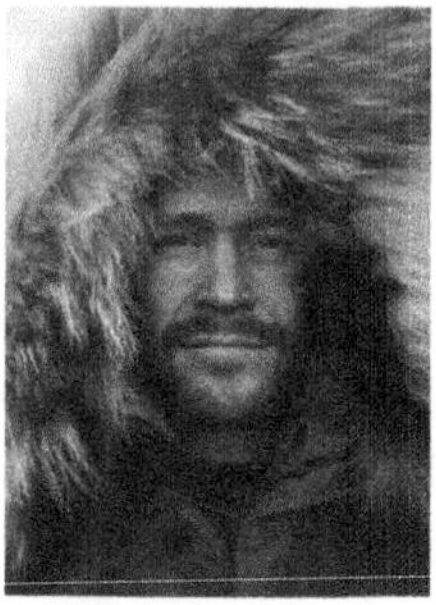

Larry Daugherty is an adventuring oncologist who holds the rank of Assistant Professor of Radiation Oncology at the Mayo Clinic. He is the co-founder of *Radiating Hope,* a nonprofit, which provides radiation oncology services in developing countries.

Dr. Daugherty received his medical degree in 2007 from University of Utah School of Medicine. He completed a residency in Radiation Oncology at Drexel University College of Medicine in Philadelphia.

In honor of his patients, he has carried Tibetan prayer flags on mountains around the world, including Everest, Denali, Kilimanjaro, Elbrus, Aconcagua, and more. He has also carried these flags on three Iditarod Trail races.

Larry lives in Eagle River, Alaska with his wife and their 5 kids.

David McHone

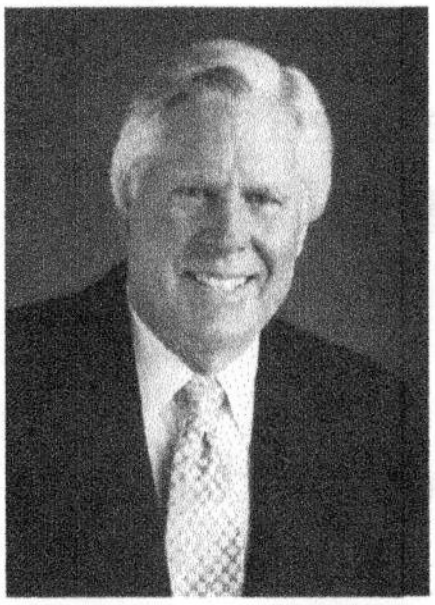

David McHone grew up in Newport Beach California and graduated from Catalina Island School For Boys in 1972. He attended the University of Puget Sound from 1972–1975, and later studied at the University of Washington Department of Fisheries, and Embryo Transplanting with Carnation Genetics in Washington State.

David was the Ranch Manager for PV Ranch Company from 1975–1983 and was awarded the California Herdsman of the Year in 1983. He has been in charge of DCM Enterprises Property Management for nearly forty years, handling assets including industrial buildings, residential housing, ranching, and aircraft hangars.

Some of David's favorite activities include golfing, skiing, snowboarding, hunting, piloting various aircraft, fishing, cowboying, wine collecting, supporting cancer causes and spending time with his wife, children and grandchildren.

Thomas J McGuire

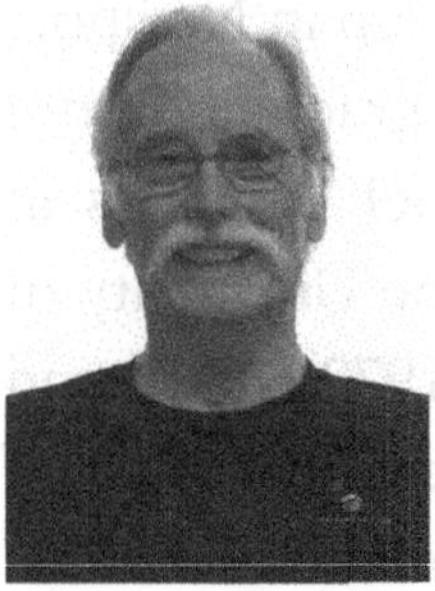

Thomas J McGuire is an advanced level Personal Trainer; certified with the American College of Sports Medicine (ACSM). His credentials include Functional Aging Specialist, and certified Qigong and Tai Chi instructor. He received his Bachelor's degree in Psychology, Physical Education and Coaching from the University of Northern Colorado. After thirty seven years of oilfield work, he started his personal training business. He is currently sponsored by the Alaska Cancer Treatment Center teaching Qigong to cancer patients. With clients ranging in age from 37–89 years, his areas of specialization include balance and strength training for stroke, arthritis, COPD and individuals with shoulder, knee, and hip injuries.

Iklim Goksel

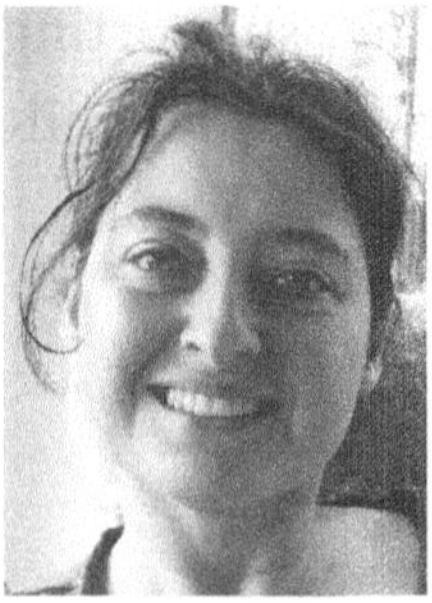

Iklim Goksel is an ethnographer and an independent scholar of Rhetoric, Gender, and Turkish Studies. She currently serves a two-year term as a policy analyst representing the state of Alaska for the National Council of Teachers of English (NCTE). She has a passionate interest in the humanities and literacy education. She is a volunteer teacher at the Alaska Literacy Program in Anchorage and works with adult immigrant and refugee populations. She earned her Bachelor's degree in English Literature from Bilkent University in Turkey, a Master's degree in Literature and Professional Writing from Eastern Michigan University, and a doctoral degree in Rhetoric from the University of Illinois at Chicago. She holds certification to teach Qigong and is currently a Tai Chi student. A native speaker of Turkish, she has also obtained professional proficiency in German and Swedish.

John and Tami Collins

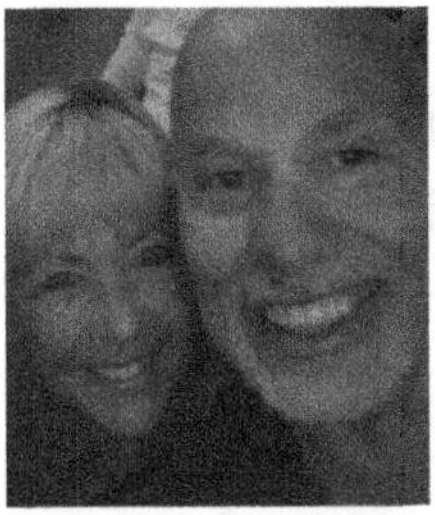

John and Tami Collins are the owners of Collins Chiropractic-A Creating Wellness Center. The focus of their office is to foster healing, growth, and repair of the body, mind, and spirit. Doctor Collins is a certified chiropractic wellness practitioner. He attained his DC from Palmer College of Chiropractic-West, and his wellness certification from the International Chiropractic Association. He specializes in teaching and coaching others through their most difficult health challenges. He begins with the new patient with one question, "What do you think the problem is and what is the solution?" This simple inquiry leads to the path back to recovered health. Doctor Collins is currently working on getting his certification as a Functional Medicine practitioner.

Tami Collins is a licensed massage therapist specializing in massage and Craniosacral therapy. She is also a certified Reiki Master. Her focus is on whole body/mind healing through her many ancient and modern techniques. After a long career in interior design specializing in the heart of the home, the kitchen, she decided to follow her own heart to be a healer. From an early age she always knew she had the gift of healing. She decided to leave her rewarding career as a kitchen designer to follow her passion of healing and health coaching.

When their noses are not buried in their array of health books, John and Tami enjoy their free time with their very mellow yellow lab Sadie, in the great Alaskan outdoors.

Torrey Smith

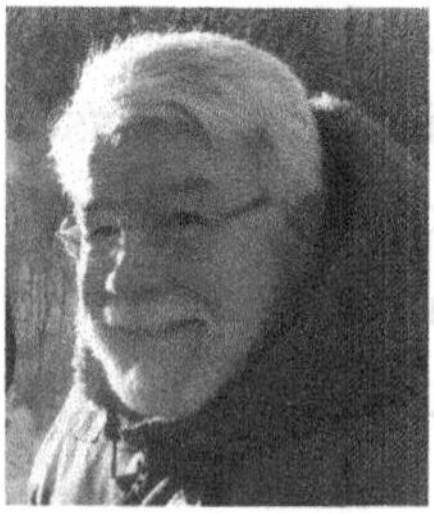

Dr. Torrey Smith ND has been a naturopathic doctor since he graduated in 1992 from NUNM. He is a life long Alaskan and has been successfully treating individuals and families in Anchorage since 1992. It has been his pleasure to help restore health and balance to thousands of great Alaskans since that time.

Dr. Smith loves to look for every possible clue to figure out the correct diagnosis and cause of disease by pouring over all the labs, tests, imaging, and symptoms that patients have had past and present to figure out how to most deeply achieve wellness. His goal is to go from frail to fantastic no matter the age or condition.

Torrey deeply cares about, and enjoys his patients, and feels incredibly lucky to spend his day with so many amazing souls. When he is not at the clinic or deep into medical journals, he loves spending time with his beautiful wife Leesha, their 6 children and 5, soon to be 6 grandchildren. His hobbies include playing guitar, gardening, hiking, and being with friends.

Matt Wilder

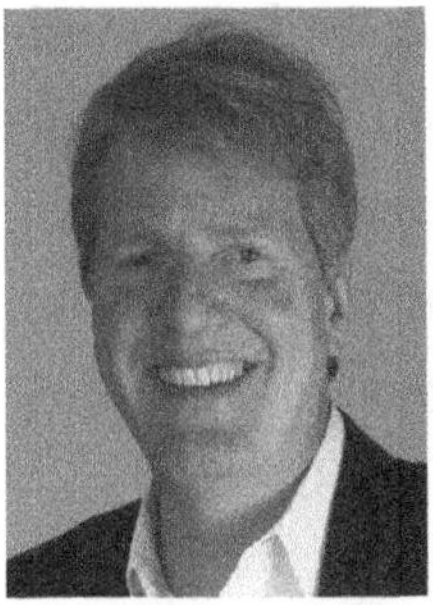

A native New Yorker, Matt has been a songwriter and recording artist since the age of 14, winning a Warner Chappell scholarship for his compositions at the age of 15. Although Matt started out as an acoustic recording artist, he began experimenting with synthesizers and sampling technology in the early 80's. He released his first two records in 1983, later signing a major label deal in 1992 with noted producer and songwriter Dan Hartmann (Tina Turner, Joe Cocker, James Brown, Steve Winwood, etc).

After Dan's untimely death in 1994, Matt started a Rock Music School which grew to over 17 bands a week, and started an Arctic Fishing lodge in Ungava, Quebec in the summers where he guided clients to several fly fishing world records, did three ESPN fishing shows, and regularly contributed to fishing publications such as *In Fisherman*, and *Fly Fisherman*.

Moving to Nashville in 2000, Matt built his own recording studio and started "Wilderside Productions" which produced demos for artists and writers from all three major labels and numerous publishing companies. Matt began teaching recording technology at Vanderbilt University in 2001, where he taught for 15 years until recently focusing full time on Remix hits.

Matt moved his production operation to Castle Recording studios in 2009. Recognizing and responding to massive changes in the recording Industry, Matt developed the concept for an automated licensing platform with co founder Sam Brooker in 2015, which turns hit songs into collaborative virtual instruments. RemixHits will hit the market late fall 2018.

Dave Nassaney

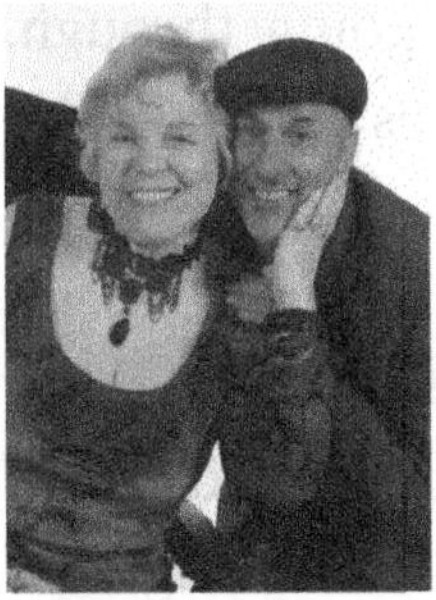

Dave Nassaney is a speaker, radio host, life-coach and best-selling author of, "It's My Life, Too! Reclaim Your Caregiver Sanity." However, his most important role is caregiver to his lovely wife, Charlene, who suffered a massive stroke 22 years ago that left her severely speech-impaired and paralyzed on the right side.

Dave has recently appeared on 24 network morning shows from Washington DC to Hawaii, and shared the stage with Suzanne Somers, at Harvard. His membership website, ***www.CaregiverDave.com***, teaches caregivers how to not only survive, but to thrive. Visit his website to get immediate practical advice and tools to stay alive, since 30% of caregivers actually die before their loved ones do, and 40%–61% (in an AARP study) felt "down, depressed and hopeless in just the past 2 weeks,"—the same symptoms that recent celebrities in the news have exhibited just before taking their own lives.

The mission of *Dave, The Caregiver's Caregiver* membership website and radio show is to help caregivers overcome adversity, the grief process, and burnout—as well as just having a safe place to rest, relax & recharge their batteries in a loving community of caring caregivers. We understand what you are going through, because we have all been there ourselves and have figured out not only how to stay alive, but to *thrive*! Dave interviews actual caregivers, who have become experts in their field and can give you actionable and practical advice to bring back the joy of caring for a loved one. If needed, Dave also offers a package of mentoring calls that will give you access to his wisdom. Learn more at ***www.CaregiverDave.com***

Thank you to the following sponsors: